A PLUM

CONQUERIN

ANNE L. PETERS, MD, is a nationally and internationally respected diabetologist, one of bestdoctors.com's Best Doctors in America, and one of the top physicians treating diabetes in America today. As professor of medicine and director of the USC Clinical Diabetes Programs, Dr. Peters treats a wide variety of patients in her two diabetes centers. One is near Beverly Hills, where she treats patients from all over the world and does clinical research on new treatments for diabetes. Her other center is in East Los Angeles, where she cares for people without health insurance. In addition, with foundation funding, she is developing a diabetes prevention and treatment program that should impact many people in Los Angeles, which has one of the largest public health systems in the world.

Dr. Peters' research has been published in leading medical journals such as *JAMA, Annals of Internal Medicine,* the *American Journal of Medicine,* and *Diabetes Care.* She has published a book on the treatment of diabetes for health care providers. As a respected expert on diabetes and its treatment she has been quoted in publications such as the *Los Angeles Times,* the *Wall Street Journal,* and the *New York Times.* The former chairperson of the American Diabetes Association Council on Health Care Delivery and Public Health, she has consulted for organizations such as Blue Cross, Wellpoint, Cigna, UniMed, and Health Net. In addition to speaking to patient groups nationally and teaching health care providers about optimal diabetes treatment, Dr. Peters has been a consultant for *E.R.,* where she made a cameo appearance in 2001, and has appeared on *Dateline,* CNN, and the Discovery Channel. She resides in Manhattan Beach, California, with her husband, Mark Harmel, her son, Max, two desert tortoises, Myrtle and Yertle, and Max-the-wonder-cat.

CONQUERING DIABETES

A Complete Program
for Prevention and Treatment

ANNE L. PETERS, MD

Photos by Mark Harmel

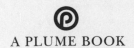

A PLUME BOOK

PLUME
Published by Penguin Group
Penguin Group (USA) Inc., 375 Hudson Street, New York, New York 10014, U.S.A.
Penguin Group (Canada), 90 Eglinton Avenue East, Suite 700, Toronto, Ontario, Canada M4P 2Y3
(a division of Pearson Penguin Canada Inc.)
Penguin Books Ltd., 80 Strand, London WC2R 0RL, England
Penguin Ireland, 25 St. Stephen's Green, Dublin 2, Ireland (a division of Penguin Books Ltd.)
Penguin Group (Australia), 250 Camberwell Road, Camberwell, Victoria 3124, Australia (a division of
Pearson Australia Group Pty. Ltd.)
Penguin Books India Pvt. Ltd., 11 Community Centre, Panchsheel Park, New Delhi – 110 017, India
Penguin Books (NZ), cnr Airborne and Rosedale Roads, Albany, Auckland 1310, New Zealand
(a division of Pearson New Zealand Ltd.)
Penguin Books (South Africa) (Pty.) Ltd., 24 Sturdee Avenue, Rosebank, Johannesburg 2196,
South Africa

Penguin Books Ltd., Registered Offices: 80 Strand, London WC2R 0RL, England

Published by Plume, a member of Penguin Group (USA) Inc. Previously published in a Hudson Street
Press edition.

First Plume Printing, April 2006
10 9 8 7 6 5 4 3 2 1

Ⓟ REGISTERED TRADEMARK—MARCA REGISTRADA

The Library of Congress has catalogued the Hudson Street Press edition as follows:
Peters, Anne L.
    Conquering diabetes : a cutting-edge, comprehensive program for prevention and treatment /
Anne Peters.
        p.   cm.
Includes index.
ISBN 1-59463-003-8 (hc.)
ISBN 0-452-28559-3 (pbk.)
1. Diabetes—Popular works.   2. Insulin resistance—Popular works.   I. Title.
RC660.4.P475   2005
616.4'62—dc22   2004026619

Printed in the United States of America
Original hardcover design by Joseph Rutt

PUBLISHER'S NOTE
Neither the publisher nor the author is engaged in rendering professional advice or services to the individual reader. The ideas, procedures, and suggestions contained in this book are not intended as a
substitute for consulting with your physician. All matters regarding your health require medical supervision. Neither the author nor the publisher shall be liable or responsible for any loss or damage al-
legedly arising from any information or suggestion in this book.

While the author has made every effort to provide accurate telephone numbers and Internet addresses
at the time of publication, neither the publisher nor the author assumes any responsibility for errors, or
for changes that occur after publication.

To my parents,
William and Virginia Peters,
with love

ACKNOWLEDGMENTS

Laurcen Rowland, my cditor and friend, conceived of the need for this book, convinced me that I could write it, and provided unending enthusiasm and support throughout the process of its creation. Without her there would be no book. Jim Levine, my agent, has patiently guided me through the unfamiliar world of nonmedical publishing and I am grateful for his encouragement and many words of wisdom.

Meg Moreta, RD, CDE, my nutritionist and Mary Rose Deraco Sosa, RN, CDE, the diabetes educator who has taught me everything I know, contributed to the writing of the nutrition and exercise chapters of this manuscript, and I am deeply grateful for their help.

This book wouldn't cxist werc it not for my wonderful patients, who teach me something new every day. They are some of the kindest and most honest people I have ever had the opportunity to know. My other teachers were those who shared their enthusiasm for knowledge and scientific inquiry during my many years of schooling. They include Mr. Kind (high school), Dr. James Donady (college), Dr. Arthur Rubenstein (medical school), and Dr. Mayer Davidson (fellowship and beyond).

Some patients help you much more than you could ever help them. Susan and Leslie Gonda are two of the dearest people I know, along with their children, Lou, Lucy, and Lorena, and the rest of the Gonda clan. From them I have learned much about survival, philanthropy, and grace. Marc Nathanson has been steadfast in his support, friendship, and advice. Anne and Arnold Kopelson have taken me under their wing and helped produce the confident-me. Barbara, Marvin, and Dana Davis, and Kelly and Robert Day have been generous and loyal supporters.

To the people I've had the pleasure to work with over the years, you have been fantastic and it is truly an honor to work with you. This list is long and includes many friends and colleagues such as Katie Arce, Bob Baravarian, Janet Bau, Dan Berger, David Boyer, Bob Briskin, Tom Buchanan, Chuck Burant, John Buse, Peter Butler, David Chan, Pejman Cohan, Ed Crandall, Jon Dann, Susan Dopart, Steve Edelman, Rob Etherington, Banning Eyre, Care Felix, Susan Fleischman, Ruth Grayless, Jeff Gutterman, Robert Henry, Paula Hunt, Lois Jovanovic, Rebecca Lyman, Jim Lower, Ruchi Mathur, Donna Miller, Flora Molina, Mike Rice, Mike Roybal, Steven Schwartz, Alan Shabo, P. K. Shah, Lauren Somma, Scott Votey, and Karol Watson.

Thanks especially to Eric Roth, for his faith in me as a person and as a doctor; to David Kendall for being the world's best adopted brother; to Howard Wisnicki for providing transcription services through his company Soft Script; to Lee Solters for generously helping me with publicity; and to Francine Kaufman for being my role model, research partner, and dear friend. And thanks to my dear now-gone grandmother Louise, who was so proud of her granddaughter doctor that she paid off my medical school loans so I could be a doctor "free and clear."

Finally, and most of all, thanks to my son Max and husband Mark, who are my strength and my solace, who see me less often than they should, but understand something of my passion to heal those who need help, and are willing to let me go.

CONTENTS

INTRODUCTION

Every day, all day, I take care of people with diabetes. My patients come in all shapes and sizes; ethnicities and ages. I see the success stories and the chronic problems. I see people I can help and, sadly, others whose complications of diabetes are too far advanced for me to impact. I see twelve-year-old girls, still innocent and on the verge of becoming young women, who are struggling to give themselves five daily insulin injections without their parents' help. I see overweight middle-aged men and women who wrestle daily with diet and exercise so they won't suffer complications of diabetes, such as blindness or life on dialysis. On the same day I see a fifty-six-year-old diabetes-related double amputee in a wheelchair I may see a seventy-six-year-old, who has had diabetes since the 1940s, who never misses his daily four-mile walk with his dog.

I know that for each and every one of these people I can minimize, possibly even prevent, diabetes complications. In many cases, I may even have prevented or delayed diabetes to begin with.

This book is an attempt to share with you the knowledge and experience I draw upon when trying to help my patients. I hope to help you, too. The information in these pages can make a big difference in your health or the health of your loved ones with diabetes. You don't need a medical degree to live well with diabetes. In fact, most doctors don't know a lot about treating diabetes. So it is up to you to gather as much knowledge as you can if you have or are at risk for diabetes.

Diabetes is growing at an epidemic rate, both worldwide and in the United States. According to the most recent statistics from the year 2000, one out of every three children born in the United States will develop diabetes in their lifetime. This number increases to one in two if the child is Latino or African American. What's traditionally been known as "adult-onset" diabetes is being diagnosed at younger and younger ages. If diabetes is diagnosed at age twenty, seventeen years of life will be lost, compared to people without diabetes. Seventeen years! It could mean you won't live long enough to retire or play with your grandkids or celebrate your thirty-fifth wedding anniversary. Even if you get diabetes later in life, say at age sixty, nine years of life will be lost. So you could miss seeing your grandkids graduate from high school and you won't be able to go on that cruise to celebrate fifty years with your spouse. But if you get good treatment for your diabetes you don't have to miss out on these and other wonderful experiences due to complications that are—and I can't stress this enough—*preventable.*

You may wonder why I am such a zealot for providing good diabetes care. I first decided to be a doctor when I was a little girl and knew, early on, that I wanted to help people with diabetes because it was an area where the need was increasing yet the number of doctors was shrinking. This is because in America insurance pays much more for the treatment of disease and relatively little for preventing it. So doctors (who, let's face it, are in business for themselves) don't want to go into a field where they can't make any money. As a result, most patients with diabetes in the United States are not able to see a diabetes specialist, and many good doctors in general practice are just too busy to provide good diabetes care. Consequently, in America in 2004, less than 10 percent of individuals with diabetes are being treated appropriately.

My career has been spent trying to teach both doctors and patients about treating and preventing diabetes. When I was a medical student at the University of Chicago, I worked with some of the most brilliant diabetes scientists in the country. I was going to be a laboratory researcher. But as I sat in the lab on the weekends, putting drops of chemicals from one little test tube into another, I realized that was not the life for me. I wanted to connect with patients, to help them apply the knowledge we already had, to help people have better, healthier lives. I knew I didn't have the patience for the slow (and very necessary) process of discovery that scientists work on every day. So after I finished my training in internal medicine at Stanford, I came to Los Angeles to study diabetes.

Los Angeles is a large, sprawling city with millions of people, many without health insurance and at very high risk for diabetes. (As I mentioned above, people of Latino or African American origin—a large portion of the L.A. population—are at very high risk for developing diabetes.) I spent my first ten years here doing clinical research, including research studies with human beings, as opposed to lab animals. As I became better known in my field, I started on what has become my life's work of designing and implementing diabetes programs—systems of care that can help thousands of people with diabetes improve their health.

I now run two diabetes centers through the University of Southern California. One is in West Los Angeles, near Beverly Hills, where I treat some of the wealthiest people in L.A. with the newest and most innovative treatments for diabetes. In West L.A. I also spend a lot of time seeing patients who want to avoid getting diabetes; we have a diabetes prevention clinic, so we can deal with this disease as early as possible, and turn it back before it starts. My other center is in East Los Angeles, in an area that is severely lacking in health care resources. None of our patients have health insurance and most are Latino. At the East L.A. Roybal Center we are able to treat people with diabetes, using simple yet effective tools. I am very proud of both of these centers and the wonderful teams of doctors, nurses, and other health care providers who work in them.

At the West and East L.A. centers we do research, both in treating and preventing diabetes. And I am now working with the County of Los Angeles to help patients throughout the region have better diabetes care. But my involvement in helping people with diabetes extends beyond Los Angeles. I travel around the country and give lectures to doctors, using my experiences in treating patients, to help them learn how to provide better care to the patients they see in their practices. I've already written a book for doctors. But the book now in your hands is written for you, the patient, because you are the one who can have the most impact on your own health.

As you read this book you'll become my patient for a while. I want to teach you the things I share with the patients I see in person so you can take care of your own diabetes and help prevent it in your loved ones who may be at risk. My first goal is to teach you how to recognize diabetes early and, ideally, how to recognize diabetes before it even starts (during a phase called prediabetes or the metabolic syndrome, which now affects an epidemic 44 million adults in this country). If diagnosed early enough many people can avoid developing diabetes; this book will describe how. The second goal is to teach you how to be an informed consumer of health care, how to work with the realities of our current health care system to achieve and maintain good health, especially with regard to diabetes. And, finally, the third goal is to explain about all of the types of diabetes and the treatments available, from both my perspective and the perspectives of my patients, some of whom have generously contributed their stories in these pages. Their experiences can help you figure out how to apply their hard-won successes to your own situation.

It is no longer enough to sit back and let your physician tell you what to do. Each of us must be empowered health care consumers. Medicine is changing rapidly, and even doctors sometimes have trouble keeping up. I hope to teach you how to ask questions that will give you control over your health, so you can fairly assess the risks and benefits before you start on any new treatment. Many people take their health for granted until they become ill, when it is often too late to make a big difference. I want you to learn what you can do early, before you have the heart attack or the diagnosis of diabetes. Or, if you have diabetes already, I will show you what you can do to avoid going blind or being attached to a dialysis machine, to keep all your limbs, foil a heart attack or stroke, and maintain an active sex life through old age.

This book is divided into four parts. There is some overlap of information between the parts, however, because in nature there are not clear delineations between the various types of diabetes. For instance, prediabetes is not considered a type of diabetes, although much of what you need to know to understand prediabetes, such as the concept of insulin resistance, is part of understanding, for example, type 2 diabetes. So it is discussed, at least in part, in the prediabetes and type 2 chapters. And the role of nutrition and exercise in the prevention and treatment of diabetes is a common theme throughout this book, so it is addressed in each part.

In the book's organization, part 1 describes the basics about the diagnosis of prediabetes and diabetes. Part 2 discusses prediabetes, which is very important for anyone who has a family member with diabetes or heart disease and may be at risk for getting diabetes in the future. The information on the prevention of diabetes is some of the newest and most cutting-edge advice in the field, and something that at the moment very few doctors know much about. Part 3 discusses type 2 diabetes, the most common form of the disease. This used to be called "adult-onset" diabetes but now we know it can happen in children even as young as three years of age. And part 4 goes into detail about type 1 diabetes, the less common form of diabetes that formerly was known as "juvenile" diabetes because it was most often diagnosed in children. These days, we know type 1 can appear at any age—I have diagnosed it in patients who are in their eighties.

The diagnosis of the types of diabetes isn't nearly as straightforward as we once thought it was, and treatment varies depending on type. So it is important that you learn how to find out what type of diabetes you have and then what you can do for it. Certain sections of the book should be read by everyone affected by diabetes, regardless of type. These include all of the chapters on nutrition (chapters 7, 10, and 17), the chapter on complications (chapter 13), and the chapter on blood glucose monitoring and hypoglycemia (chapters 10 and 15).

I hope that this book functions as the motivational resource you need to help you take action in preventing or treating diabetes. At the very least it should help you understand which questions you should ask your health care team and how you can monitor your progress and maintain your health. I know how hard it is to find the time to take care of your health, especially when you are busy or feel fine. But think of how hard it is to drag yourself to the doctor when you feel ill—it takes twice the energy than when you feel healthy. So go early, before you feel sick.

Prediabetes and diabetes are disorders that are fairly easy to follow—as you'll see, much of monitoring diabetes is based on numbers, whether for your blood sugar, cholesterol, or blood pressure levels. And with a little effort you can learn what these numbers mean and follow them yourself. The only thing to avoid is feeling discouraged or judged. I often hear patients use the word "failure"; I refuse to let people use it in my clinic. We have therapies that allow us to treat prediabetes and diabetes successfully and if one approach doesn't work we can add or switch to another. And, as you'll read in the essays my patients wrote for this book, positive outcomes are possible. I want to help you get there, too. Diabetes is manageable, but you must take the initiative and make the effort to manage it.

Through this book we are now a team working together to help you stay healthy. The good news is you're not in this alone.

PART ONE

UNDERSTANDING THE DIAGNOSIS

ONE

DIAGNOSIS OF DIABETES AND PREDIABETES

You've just been told by your doctor that your blood sugar level is "a touch too high." You've been given these little blue pills to take and assured that "everything will be okay." The problem is, you don't feel like everything will be okay. You are overwhelmed and confused. You desperately want to avoid the fate that befell your aunt Sylvia, as she struggled with her dialysis treatments and ended up dying after a month in a cardiac intensive care unit. You've watched your mother fret over your father as he reaches for one more piece of bread or a second helping of dessert because she's afraid of what it will do to his diabetes. You think that you, too, will have to stop eating all of your favorite foods and will never be able to enjoy life in the same way again. You worry that you will go blind; the fact that your eyes are blurry from your recently elevated blood sugar levels only confirms this fear. Finally, you are sure that the recent tingling in your toes (also caused by your suddenly high blood sugar levels) means nerve damage and a possible future amputation.

So what do you do? Is there *anything* you can do? Yes, there is.

You learn. You learn everything possible about diabetes. You turn yourself into an expert. You learn how you can help your father, yourself, and perhaps your children. You learn how you can treat and even prevent diabetes. You learn that it is completely within your power to alter the course of this disease. Diabetes doesn't have a cure—yet. But it can be tamed and managed, *if* you understand who and what is at risk and how best to deal with all the related issues.

PREDIABETES AND DIABETES DEFINED

The first thing you need to learn is the difference between prediabetes and diabetes. Knowing what prediabetes and diabetes are, and understanding the similarities and differences between them, makes it easier to find out if you have one of these conditions. Prediabetes means that you don't yet have diabetes, but if you do nothing you may develop type 2 diabetes in the future. The biggest worry with prediabetes is an increased risk for heart disease, even if diabetes never develops. When you have prediabetes you have something called insulin resistance. This means that your body doesn't respond correctly to the insulin your body makes. Your body then has to make more and more insulin to keep your blood sugar levels in the normal range. When you have insulin resistance, other abnormalities of fat and blood pressure occur that can clog your arteries with plaque. So when I talk about treating prediabetes I am talking about preventing both diabetes and heart disease. This condition (and its associated disorder known as the metabolic syndrome, or syndrome X) is very common; more than 44 million Americans have it.

Diabetes, which is an abnormality of blood sugar levels, is classified by three distinct types. Type 2 is the most common and is the type of diabetes people get if their prediabetes is not treated. Type 1 diabetes is the form of diabetes for which patients must take insulin shots for the rest of their lives. The third type is gestational diabetes, which is a form of type 2 diabetes that can occur during pregnancy. When I treat patients with type 1 and type 2 diabetes, I work with them to bring blood sugar, blood pressure, and cholesterol levels into the normal range. This helps lower their risk for heart disease and stroke (just as in patients with prediabetes) as well as the risk for blindness, kidney failure, and amputation.

When you are first diagnosed with prediabetes or diabetes you need to find health care providers who can give you the education and treatment that you need. Later in the book (chapter 3) I will describe how to find help, and who can give it. What is most important to realize right now is that we can do something about prediabetes and diabetes. Having these conditions isn't a death sentence. Think of them instead as an opportunity to take control, to have a longer, healthier life. Many of the diabetes management skills I hope to teach you in this book will make you (actually *anyone*) healthier overall. Fixing one part of your health (for instance, increasing the fiber in your diet to help lower blood sugar and cholesterol levels) can also affect another area (such as lowering the risk for colon cancer). Treating diabetes is treating your well-being overall.

THE RISKS FOR PREDIABETES AND TYPE 2 DIABETES

Prediabetes can turn into type 2 diabetes, which means they share the same spectrum of illness. Both involve blood sugar level, an important measure for anyone at risk for either condition to know. The higher your blood sugar, the greater your chances of having diabetic problems (which we call "complications") in the future. A normal fasting (before eating) blood sugar level is less than 100 milligrams per decaliter (mg/dl). Anything sustained above 100 mg/dl is considered abnormal. If your fasting blood sugar level is between 100 to 125 mg/dl we say you have prediabetes. If your blood sugar level rises above 125 you have diabetes. Your goal, then, is to bring your blood sugar levels down to as close to normal as possible and keep them there for the rest of your life.

There are several reasons why a normal blood sugar level is so important. First, if your blood sugar levels are high over a long period of time (more than ten years) you are at risk for developing the complications of diabetes. The most serious include diabetic eye disease (a cause of blindness), nerve damage (which can lead to amputation of your feet or legs as well as disorders of the functioning of your intestines, bladder, stomach, and heart, and also cause impotence), and kidney damage (which can cause kidney failure and require dialysis or kidney transplant). High blood sugar levels often are associated with high levels of fat in the blood (called cholesterol and triglyceride). These can double or quadruple your risk for heart disease or stroke. Finally, patients with prediabetes and diabetes are also at a very high risk for having high blood pressure, which is another key factor in heart attacks and strokes.

The questions below list all of the risk factors for both prediabetes and type 2 diabetes combined. The two are fairly indistinguishable, because a risk for one is the same as the risk for the other. But the more risk factors you have, the more likely you are to have prediabetes or type 2 diabetes. However, you can have prediabetes or diabetes without any of these risk factors. When studies for diabetes featuring questionnaires have been conducted they weren't terribly reliable indicators of who does and doesn't have prediabetes or diabetes. The best way to find out is to ask your doctor for a fasting blood sugar test and then to follow your blood sugar level every year to be sure it remains normal.

RISK FACTOR PROFILE

Any "yes" answer increases your risk for prediabetes or type 2 diabetes.

1. Are you overweight, particularly with most of your weight around your center?

2. Are you all or partially of African American, Latino, American Indian, Asian, or Pacific Islander origin?

3. Are you older than forty-five?

4. Do you have a family history of type 2 diabetes (parent, grandparent, or child)?

5. Do you have high blood pressure?

6. Have you had a heart attack?

7. Do you have a triglyceride (fat in the blood) level greater than 150 mg/dl?

8. Do you have a good cholesterol (high-density lipoprotein or HDL cholesterol) level that is too low, which means less than 40 mg/dl in a male or less than 50 mg/dl in a female?

9. Have you had gestational diabetes or a baby weighing more than 9 pounds in the past?

10. Have you ever been told you had impaired glucose tolerance or prediabetes in the past?

11. Do you have polycystic ovarian syndrome (PCOS) (a specifi-
    cally female form of insulin resistance, discussed in chapter 6)?

12. Do you rarely or never exercise?

**Insulin resistance can appear before any rise
in blood sugar levels.**

You can have insulin resistance before you have any elevation in
blood sugar levels, and before you are diagnosed with prediabetes
(a blood sugar level between 100 and 125 mg/dl). This is the limbo
of the metabolic syndrome or syndrome X. The patients I see with
this syndrome usually are people who have a mother or father with
diabetes who want to know their risk for getting diabetes. Their
blood sugar level may be normal (less than 100 mg/dl), but they
have extra fat around the middle, an elevation in triglyceride levels,
and a reduction in their HDL (good) cholesterol level. I immediately suspect these patients have insulin resistance. If I measured
their insulin level, a test not currently recommended to diagnose
insulin resistance (except in research studies), I expect to find that
it is elevated. This means that these patients are insulin resistant.
Their bodies are making extra insulin to compensate for their resistance and to keep their blood sugar levels normal. I will discuss this
syndrome in more detail in part 2, but it's important to note that
people who have early insulin resistance should still know that they
are at risk. It is best they follow the same strategy for preventing diabetes and heart disease as those who have prediabetes.

DIAGNOSING PREDIABETES AND DIABETES

How do you know if you have prediabetes or diabetes? Most people
who have prediabetes or diabetes have no symptoms. So let's go
back to the risk factor profile we did. Knowing your family medical
history is valuable. If you have a parent or child or grandparent

with diabetes you are at risk for having diabetes yourself. Certain ethnic groups—African American, American Indian, Latino, Asian, Pacific Islanders—have increased risk for diabetes. If you are a member of one of these ethnic groups your risk for diabetes goes up one and a half to two times more than someone from a different ethnic background. I also see a lot of prediabetes and diabetes in people who come from Eastern Europe (for example, the former East Germany, Poland, and Hungary) as well as from the countries of the former Soviet Union.

The risk for prediabetes and diabetes starts with your genes. In an environment where food is plentiful and exercise is lacking, certain genes (called "thrifty genes") cause prediabetes and diabetes. Researchers think these genes helped our ancestors survive through periods of famine by aiding the body with the storage of fat. This fat was stored in the center of the body, close to all of the internal organs. From there it could quickly be metabolized to feed the liver and increase the production of sugar, giving the brain enough fuel to function. But if these genes, designed to hoard energy for survival, are fed too much food that isn't burned off through exercise, they create a metabolic imbalance and cause prediabetes and diabetes.

The risk for prediabetes and diabetes starts with your genes.

Many things beyond genes can cause insulin resistance to get worse. Getting older makes us all more insulin resistant. This is why type 2 diabetes used to be called "adult-onset" diabetes. We now know that it can occur in children as well. In fact, as children are becoming more overweight and less active, their genes for insulin resistance are creating diabetes earlier and earlier. However, prediabetes and diabetes are still more common in adults, especially as they age, exercise less, and put on additional pounds. Most Americans gain 2 pounds of weight each year and this gradual increase in body fat slowly but surely makes us more likely to get diabetes, as becoming overweight makes our cells less responsive to insulin. Extra fat begins to act like toxic glue, sending out signals to the muscles, liver, pancreas, and other organs that interfere with their normal functioning. This action is not completely understood, but it *does* happen.

Lack of exercise also increases the risk for diabetes. Our bodies were meant to be physically active. Using our muscles increases their demand for fuel and this increases their ability to respond to insulin. Many studies show that regular exercise helps to more efficiently burn fat and sugar calories and keep our insulin resistance at a lower level. The problem with exercise, though, is that its beneficial effects don't last for more than a few days. So to optimize metabolic efficiency, we need to exercise at least five days a week.

Like prediabetes, diabetes often has no symptoms. If you're high on the risk profile scale, it is even more important for you to ask your doctor to check your fasting blood sugar level every year. Do not believe your doctor if he or she tells you that your blood sugar is fine. Ask for the number and if it is above 100 mg/dl you need to find someone who can diagnose and treat your prediabetes or diabetes. I have had many, many patients whose physicians told them not to worry when they had blood sugar levels of 140 mg/dl or even more. They were going untreated, at risk for complications, because their physicians did not appropriately respond to elevated blood sugar levels.

Like prediabetes, diabetes often has no symptoms.

Remember, *it is most common for people with diabetes and prediabetes to show no symptoms.* Even if symptoms of diabetes are present they tend to be subtle at first, becoming more dramatic over time. In patients who do have symptoms, the most frequent complaint I hear is that they are getting up more often at night to urinate. This is called nocturia. When extra sugar in the blood is leaking out into the urine more water is drawn into the urine. This increases the amount of urine and the frequency with which one has to go to the bathroom. (When this happens during the day it is called polyuria.) The extra fluid lost in the urine may make you feel an increase in thirst. People will tell me that they were craving large quantities of cola, orange juice, or water in the month before they were diagnosed. This thirst is the body's attempt to replace the fluids lost in excess urination due to high sugar levels.

Sometimes people lose a lot of weight before they are diagnosed with diabetes. I have seen people who look like they are wasting away because they don't know they have diabetes and are running around with incredibly high blood sugar levels. The reason you lose weight when your blood sugar levels are very high is because all the sugar, the fuel for the body, is on the outside of the cells instead of being pushed by insulin to the inside, where it is needed for energy. These patients are so resistant to the action of insulin and make so little insulin on their own that their blood sugar levels, with nothing to keep them in check, inevitably rise. Someone in this condition may eat thousands of calories per day, but their body can't process the calories it is taking in. In other words, the person begins to starve. They also can become severely dehydrated because, as mentioned above, their bodies try to flush out the extra sugar in their blood by putting additional water into their urine.

High blood sugar levels also seem to make people fatigued.

People with high sugar levels often seem prone to infections. And when they get infections they don't recover or heal as quickly as usual. This is because high sugar levels inhibit the body's ability to fight infection—the white blood cells, which are the infection-fighting cells, don't work as well when sugar levels are high. Women who are getting diabetes will often complain of frequent vaginal yeast infections because it seems that yeasts are particularly fond of a high sugar environment.

High blood sugar levels also seem to make people fatigued. Most likely this is because their cells aren't being fed enough sugar from the bloodstream, so they lack the energy they need to function optimally. It's not that they want to sleep all the time; it's just that they feel too tired to do anything that requires extra effort. I think that sometimes the increase in blood sugar levels happens so gradually that people don't notice how tired they really are. Once blood sugar levels come down, my patients often say that they have more energy than they have had in years.

Another common complaint that people have when their blood sugar levels rise above normal is blurry vision. This isn't the same as diabetic retinopathy, in which the back of the eyeball becomes damaged by chronically elevated blood sugars. Instead, this is a problem affecting the lens in the front of the eye and may be most noticeable even as blood sugar levels are brought down to normal. Sugar tends to stay in the lens longer than it does in the blood. This imbalance causes the lens to change shape and distort vision as fluid moves in and out of it. This change is not permanent, and unlike other diabetic eye damage, it is not serious. But it can take a month or two to go away and often causes a lot of concern because it can interfere with reading and doing everyday work.

Other medical problems can be indicators of prediabetes or diabetes. These include heart attack or having elevated fats (cholesterol and triglycerides) in the blood. High blood pressure is another contributing factor. If you are female, you need to be aware of polycystic ovarian syndrome (PCOS), which is a form of insulin resistance that leads to irregular menstrual cycles and infertility. Having had gestational diabetes (diabetes during pregnancy, which is discussed in chapter 6 in more detail) also puts you at increased risk for diabetes. Finally, if you notice that you have a darkening of the skin under your arms or around the back of your neck you could have something called acanthosis nigricans. This mysterious condition causes your skin to become pigmented as a reaction to the high insulin levels that accompany insulin resistance. It is not harmful by itself, but can be a sign of an internal metabolic imbalance.

How and When to Get Tested for Prediabetes and Diabetes

If you have any of the symptoms of diabetes mentioned above, particularly excessive thirst or urination and weight loss, you should see your physician immediately. Not to alarm you, but this is considered a medical emergency. If you are having trouble drinking enough water to control your thirst or are vomiting, you should not wait to hear from or visit your doctor. Go to an emergency room or an urgent care center right away. You may need to be given intravenous fluids and even admitted to a hospital. Fortunately, such severe early symptoms are rare, but must be quickly investigated if they occur.

Anyone with any of the risk factors I listed, even if they don't
have symptoms, should have a screening test for prediabetes and
diabetes. This is especially important for those over forty-five or
with a family history of diabetes. A screening test can be done at
any age. For example, in Los Angeles, where prediabetes and diabetes is being found in high school students, we are testing children as young as ten years old. If your risk for diabetes is high you
may need to be screened every year. For patients with a lower risk,
every three years is sufficient. The specific recommendations for
screening are not concrete. As a guideline, however, if you have
two or three of the prediabetes and diabetes risk factors, you probably should be tested annually.

A screening test can be done at any age.

The Blood Tests for Diagnosing Prediabetes and Diabetes

The tests for prediabetes and diabetes involve simple blood work
that your primary care physician can do. You need to have your
fasting blood sugar level determined and a lipid panel (good and
bad cholesterol as well as triglyceride levels) measured. Fasting
means having nothing to eat or drink (except water) for about ten
hours before the blood sample is taken. Twelve hours is best if you
can wait that long. Usually, the blood is taken first thing in the
morning. If you are having a fasting blood test done and will have
to wait for a while before you get back home or to work, you may
want to bring some food to eat after the blood is drawn to avoid
getting too hungry.

You can also have your blood sugar level measured at a health
fair or other public event, but often the results aren't as complete
or as accurate as those your physician can provide. Be sure that in
either case you obtain copies of your laboratory reports. That way
you can keep track of any changes over time and you can use them
to compare to the values specified in this book.

Fasting blood sugar levels fall into three categories. If your level
is above 125 mg/dl you have diabetes. If it is 100 to 125 mg/dl you

have prediabetes, which means you are at risk for getting diabetes as well as heart disease. If it is less than 100 mg/dl you may be normal, although you still can have an increased risk for heart disease.

If you are having symptoms of diabetes, such as excessive thirst and urination, and your random (not fasting—taken any time of day) blood sugar level is above 200 mg/dl, you almost certainly have diabetes. This is not the most common way to diagnose diabetes, as most people won't have the symptoms to indicate a test should be done. Testing for an increased blood sugar level is very simple—your fingertip can be poked for a sample, or blood can be drawn from your vein. Either way a simple, accurate test can be done.

People used to be tested for diabetes with an oral glucose tolerance test, which meant giving patients a very sweet type of cola or orange drink after the blood sugar level was taken, then measuring another level two hours later. This type of test isn't done very often these days because it takes too long and isn't terribly accurate. Occasionally, a doctor will order it to help diagnose very subtle abnormalities of glucose metabolism. Personally, I almost never use glucose tolerance tests, except in pregnancy, when they are done routinely at 25 to 28 weeks to determine whether or not the mother has gestational diabetes. I prefer to use the fasting glucose level to help me understand what is going on because it is a simple test for the patient and, in my experience, provides accurate information.

Testing for an increased blood sugar level is very simple—your fingertip can be poked for a sample, or blood can be drawn from your vein.

Another number that you should know about is called a "glycated hemoglobin level," "hemoglobin A1C level," or simply "A1C." The term A1C is the new official term (and the one I'll use) based on the recommendations of the American Diabetes Association and other organizations. The reason for the change is that people were confusing the word "hemoglobin" (a measure of how many red blood cells you have) with "hemoglobin A1C," which is a measure of how much sugar you have attached to your red blood cells. It was felt that taking away the word "hemoglobin" altogether would make it easier for people to focus on the fact that this is a test of glucose levels, not red blood cell mass. To say it, you say the letter "A," then "one," then "C." It may be listed as something else (one of the older terms) on a laboratory report, but it should always have A1C (or A₁c) in the name.

A1C is a measure of the average sugar level in your blood over the past three months. Three months is the life span of a red blood cell, so the A1C can change over a test period. If your A1C level starts to go up it is a sign that you might need a change in your diabetes medications. When we test you in the office or when you test your blood sugar level at home, that reading is just one measurement in time compared to the numerous up and down fluctuations of your blood sugar level as you go through a day. The A1C test averages all of your blood sugar changes over the last three months and the resulting level provides a relative correlation to your risk for having complications of diabetes. Obviously, you always want to keep your blood sugar level as close to normal as possible. If your A1C is 4 to 6 percent, you are considered to be in the normal range; above normal almost certainly indicates prediabetes or diabetes. My goal when treating diabetes is to test my patients' A1C level every three months. I try to keep their A1C results well below 7 percent and as close to 6 percent as possible. That way, they are at the lowest known risk for getting the complications of diabetes.

A1C is a measure of the average sugar level in your blood over the past three months.

Initially, you should have the fasting blood sugar test done twice to make the diagnosis of diabetes. Many times this is not done—especially when the blood sugar level is very high. However, as a doctor I have enough skepticism about any laboratory test to want to do it a second time. That way I'm sure I'm not giving someone a wrong diagnosis.

Often a nonfasting, or random, blood sugar level will be measured as part of a blood panel. This is done because we tend to order "panels" of blood tests—groups of chemistries that cost less if the machine measures an entire series of things as opposed to an individual test. Someone without diabetes never has a blood sugar level above 140 mg/dl—*never,* not even one hour after eating twenty pancakes with syrup. Sometimes when I find blood sugar in a patient that is 250 mg/dl, the patient says, "Don't worry, I just ate a doughnut." But I *do* worry. *Regardless of what you've eaten, a blood sugar level above 140 mg/dl is not normal and needs to be checked out.*

Regardless of what you've eaten, a blood sugar level above 140 mg/dl is not normal and needs to be checked out.

Far too often I've seen patients with high random blood sugar levels whose conditions have gone untreated and unevaluated for years and years. Don't be one of these people. Any suspicion of high blood sugar level should be assessed by having your fasting blood sugar level measured. It's better to know if you have diabetes or prediabetes. Even if the test shows only a risk for diabetes you'll know you should maintain a healthy weight and exercise regularly. Then have your blood sugar tested again every year and track the blood sugar numbers to be sure they stay in the normal range (less than 100 mg/dl). If they don't, treatments such as better nutrition, increased physical activity, and a variety of oral medications can keep you healthy.

At the same time you get your fasting blood sugar level tested you should ask for a fasting lipid panel. You will want to know the following levels: triglycerides, total cholesterol, LDL (bad) cholesterol, and HDL (good) cholesterol. If the triglycerides are above 150 mg/dl and the HDL is below 50 (if you are female) or 40 (if you are male) you may be at risk for heart disease and prediabetes or diabetes.

Understanding the Test Numbers

When you have diabetes or even prediabetes you quickly become fluent with test numbers because you may be checking your own sugar levels several times each day. Reading and interpreting these numbers becomes second nature. The numbers in the chart below are strictly to help you make sense of test results.

TABLE 1

Test	Value	Condition
Fasting (prebreakfast) blood sugar level	Less than 100 mg/dl	Usually this is normal
Fasting (prebreakfast) blood sugar level	100 to 125 mg/dl	Prediabetes
Fasting (prebreakfast) blood sugar level	Greater than 125 mg/dl	Diabetes
A1C level	Less than 6 percent	Usually normal or prediabetes
A1C level	6 percent or more	Prediabetes or diabetes (almost always diabetes if greater than 7 percent)
Random (any time of day) blood sugar level	140 to 200 mg/dl	Possibly diabetes
Random (any time of day) blood sugar level with symptoms of thirst, excessive urination, weight loss	More than 200 mg/dl	Diabetes

AFTER A DIAGNOSIS OF PREDIABETES OR DIABETES

If you are diagnosed with diabetes or prediabetes your world changes and you will be full of conflicting feelings. But no matter what you are feeling or thinking, don't panic. And, equally important, don't go into denial. Diabetes can be treated and managed, even if it can't yet (I emphasize *yet*) be cured. If you pay attention to your diabetes, learn what you need to do to stay healthy, and find the right health care, you will be absolutely fine. We can't make the disease go away, but we can do a lot to prevent any possible complications and show you how to live a life not much different from the one you now have. The earlier you get help, the better off you will be.

Most people initially are treated for their diabetes by their general doctor—often an internist or a family practitioner. Many general doctors think that they can treat diabetes adequately and although they may possess the knowledge to treat diabetes, many don't have enough time to treat diabetes well. I think that anyone who has type 1 diabetes—and most people with type 2 diabetes who require insulin—should be followed by an endocrinologist. An endocrinologist is someone who is trained first in internal medicine and then in endocrinology, which is the study of hormones. Some endocrinologists treat mostly nondiabetes hormones, such as those from the thyroid or the adrenal gland. A few, like me, specialize in diabetes, which involves the hormone insulin. Although I can treat all endocrine problems, my focus is on diabetes.

Unfortunately there aren't enough endocrinologists to go around. Most are located in big cities, near universities. They are very rarely found in rural areas, as there are fewer patients there who need them. But don't despair if you can't find an endocrinologist. You may be able to find a diabetes educator who can help you in concert with your primary care doctor. And this book will help you learn what you need to do to stay healthy and live long with diabetes.

Once Your Treatment Begins

At first you may feel like your entire life has been taken over by diabetes. You'll have lots of appointments, quite possibly you'll need to learn a new way to eat, and you will have to test your blood sugar levels throughout the day by pricking your finger and putting a drop of blood on a strip that slides into a glucose meter. To a certain extent it is like going back to school because learning will have to be a conscious effort and it will require some discipline. Don't despair, however, because if you put in the time up front and learn how to manage your diabetes, it will become second nature. Sure, it will always be a problem you wish you didn't have, but it *will* become less of a burden. If you manage your diabetes with intelligence and diligence, it becomes less overwhelming and more of an annoyance that occasionally impinges on your spontaneity.

Gary Hall Jr., an Olympic swimmer and a friend of mine who has type 1 diabetes, tests his blood sugar levels up to ten times per day when he is training. He says that testing has become as routine as brushing his teeth—it is just something he does. That is what I wish for you—access to the training and knowledge you need so that taking care of your prediabetes or diabetes becomes a natural part of your existence. Many of my patients—people I am privileged to know—do beautifully with their diabetes. I want this book to give you the confidence and the skills to do every bit as well as they do.

Facing prediabetes and diabetes may be overwhelming at first, but trust me, it will become easier with time. Your confusion will gradually disappear and you will learn how to adopt new, healthier patterns. In some ways diabetes may help you become healthier than ever. Depending on whether you have prediabetes, type 1, or type 2 diabetes, your treatment will differ a bit. But before we get to my advice on how to proceed once diabetes is diagnosed, let's step back and I'll give you a brief overview of the forms of the disease and the potential complications associated with it.

....

TWO

THE DIABETES SPECTRUM

By now you know that there are two primary types of diabetes, type 1 and type 2, and that gestational diabetes can occur in pregnant women. Prediabetes, as mentioned earlier, can become full-blown diabetes, but is not considered diabetes even though it can contribute to many of the same major health risks. It usually starts ten to fifteen years before it turns into type 2 diabetes. All of these forms of the disease are discussed in greater detail in the later sections of this book. What follows in this chapter, though, is a survey of the diabetes spectrum in all its shades. By being aware right up front of the various aspects of diabetes—from presumed causes through potential complications—you will be better able to understand this book and use the information it contains to your advantage.

TYPE 2 DIABETES

Type 2 diabetes occurs in approximately 15 million Americans, although one-third of the people who have it don't know that they do. We used to call this "adult-onset" diabetes because we thought that only young people got type 1 diabetes and older people got type 2 diabetes. Now we know that you can get either type of diabetes at any age. Children as young as two years old are developing type 2 diabetes, so we no longer can define it as an adult phenomenon.

Most people who have this type of diabetes are overweight and nearly everyone has a family member who has type 2 diabetes or heart disease. It is much more common in people who have ancestors who are American Indian, Latino, African American, Asian, or from the Pacific Islands. In my experience ancestors from Eastern Europe also increase the risk for type 2 diabetes. However, it's important to note that not being in one of these high-risk ethnic groups doesn't mean that you are automatically immune to the disease.

People with type 2 diabetes always have two conditions—insulin resistance and insulin deficiency.

Insulin resistance is a concept that all people with diabetes must understand. When the body does not respond normally to the insulin it makes, it requires more and more insulin to maintain normal blood sugar levels. Over time, the necessity of producing all this extra insulin puts a terrible strain on the insulin-producing (beta) cells in your pancreas. Eventually these cells can't make enough insulin, insulin production falls off, and you develop *insulin deficiency*. Then blood sugar levels can increase dramatically. This dual problem of insulin resistance plus insulin deficiency is what causes type 2 diabetes.

It is possible that you can be very insulin resistant yet not have diabetes. For instance, you could weigh 400 pounds, but if you don't have the genes for diabetes your pancreas will just keep making large amounts of insulin and your blood sugar levels will stay normal. If you happen to have the genes for diabetes, for reasons we don't completely understand, your beta cells stop making enough insulin and your blood sugar levels increase. When we look at the beta cells of patients with type 2 diabetes they look like they are filled with pink chewing gum (a substance called amyloid) instead of like healthy insulin-secreting cells. The amyloid clogs the beta cells, thereby reducing the efficiency of the pancreas to produce the insulin you need to balance your blood sugar and stay healthy.

Overweight patients with type 2 diabetes can often be helped by weight loss and exercise alone. Losing weight makes the body more sensitive again to insulin, so blood sugar levels fall. If you are at risk for diabetes and can avoid gaining weight as you age, that is the best strategy of all; it is far harder to lose weight than to prevent weight gain. If lifestyle changes don't work, there are a number of different types of oral medications for treating type 2 diabetes. You may need one single type of pill or a combination of pills. If oral medications don't work, insulin injections are added to make the treatment more effective.

Overweight patients with type 2 diabetes can often be helped by weight loss and exercise alone.

TYPE 1 DIABETES AND LADA

Having type 1 diabetes means your insulin-secreting (beta) cells have shut down completely and your body no longer produces any insulin. Once in this state, you must take insulin shots. This type of diabetes is much less common than type 2 diabetes—about 1.5 million Americans have it. Type 1 diabetes is a form of autoimmune disease, like lupus and rheumatoid arthritis, where your own antibodies attack the cells that secrete insulin. In other words, your body is basically destroying parts of itself. This sounds slightly worse than it is. Still, your immune system is seriously malfunctioning. Normally, when an "invader," such as a virus, enters your body, your immune system makes antibodies against it that surround and kill the infection. But in order to do this, your body must have a sophisticated system for determining what is abnormal and what is "self."

In type 1 diabetes (and in other diseases like lupus and rheumatoid arthritis) the body starts to make antibodies to its own beta cells. This process is thought to happen both because of genes (some sort of inherited predisposition to this process) and an environmental process (maybe a toxin, another virus, or an allergen) that makes the immune system misfire. Once your body starts making antibodies to your beta cells, they begin dying. At some point you'll have too few living cells to make enough insulin to keep your blood

sugar levels in the normal range. Once glucose levels start to rise—
and stay high—you will be diagnosed with type 1 diabetes. The only
known effective treatment for type 1 diabetes is replacing the
body's insulin with outside insulin through daily injections.

Type 1 diabetes often happens much more suddenly than type
2 diabetes, which can smolder, slowly developing over years and
years. In children, type 1 diabetes seems to come on fast; kids who
develop diabetes will immediately need to be treated with insulin.
In adults, though, type 1 diabetes may come on more gradually. My
oldest patient with newly diagnosed type 1 (formerly called "juvenile" diabetes) is eighty-seven years old—clearly not a kid anymore,
except perhaps in spirit.

---

*The only known effective treatment for type 1 diabetes
is replacing the body's insulin with outside insulin
through daily injections.*

This kind of adult-onset type 1 diabetes is called latent autoimmune diabetes of the adult (LADA). Some people call this type
1.5 diabetes, but I prefer the term LADA since it better explains
what it is. People with LADA are often mistakenly thought to have
type 2 diabetes and are treated with pills. However, the pills don't
work very well (because they are made for treating a different type
of diabetes). Insulin is almost always required.

....

"I thought type 1 diabetes only happened in childhood."

Maria is a fifty-six-year-old woman, active in her community and
full of energy and spirit. Having type 1 diabetes, misdiagnosed
as type 2 at first, really perplexed her because she couldn't
quite stabilize herself. Now that she knows what type of diabetes
she has, she has been able to control her diabetes so much better, and management of the disease is no longer the struggle it
once was for her.

*My diagnosis of diabetes came like a bolt out of the blue. No one in
my family ever had diabetes. My family comes from Northern Europe*

and Great Britain and although a few family members have developed heart disease and cancer as they got older, none have had diabetes. I thought that diabetes was something that happened if you were overweight or if your parents had it. And although I have always struggled a bit with my weight, I did not consider myself fat or at risk for diabetes.

I went to my doctor because I was feeling thirsty and going to the bathroom more frequently, especially at night. My doctor measured my blood sugar level and said it was way too high. He told me I had diabetes. So he put me on pills. Many different pills. The more pills I tried, the worse I felt. I learned to test my blood sugar levels and measured several times per day. I found that I could lower my blood sugar levels by eating a very limited diet, but overall I felt that I was struggling and struggling and getting nowhere. One day my sugar level would be 90 and the next day it would be 300. It made no sense.

One day I happened to run into someone who was a diabetes specialist for children. She said she'd heard I'd been diagnosed with diabetes. When I told her that yes, I had type 2 diabetes, she was aghast. She insisted that I had type 1 diabetes and needed to see a specialist right away. She thought this just from looking at me. I told her that I thought type 1 diabetes only happened in childhood, and she told me that wasn't true anymore and I needed a second opinion.

I was somewhat reluctant to go to see a new doctor, because I liked my doctor and he practiced near my house, but I needed answers. To make a long story short, I went to see Dr. Peters. She did blood tests and found out that I had LADA, or type 1 diabetes. She said that what I needed was insulin shots, not pills. And although it has been a bit difficult getting used to the routine of the shots, I felt immediately better once I was off the oral diabetes medication. And finally having an answer as to why my diabetes was so tough to treat was quite a relief. I wasn't quite so frustrated anymore and now I finally have good control of my blood sugars.

....

GESTATIONAL DIABETES

Another type of diabetes can occur during pregnancy. This is called gestational diabetes or GDM. In a way, this is a form of type 2 diabetes because when a woman is pregnant she becomes more resistant to the effects of insulin. This actually makes sense because her body wants to make sure the developing baby has enough sugar to sustain it and grow. So the hormones associated with pregnancy can, in some cases, cause enough insulin resistance to bring on *temporary* type 2 diabetes. Most women are screened for gestational diabetes during pregnancy, because if it occurs and is missed it can adversely affect the baby. It is significant to note that 50 percent of women who have had gestational diabetes develop type 2 diabetes at some point later in life. So if you have had gestational diabetes you must be certain to be tested every year following pregnancy to be sure you haven't developed another type of diabetes.

TABLE 2

Type of Diabetes Mellitus	Who Gets It	Tests for It	Treatment
Type 2	All ages, although mostly adults; most common type of diabetes	Fasting blood sugar; no special test needed	Diet and exercise, pills, insulin as needed
Type 1— children	Kids	Fasting sugar; antibody tests can confirm it (anti-islet cell antibodies)	Insulin
Type 1— adults (also called LADA)	Adults of any age	Fasting sugar; anti-GAD antibodies confirm it*	Mostly insulin
Gestational	Pregnant women	Oral glucose tolerance	Diet and exercise, insulin

*See page 258.

FACING THE FACTS EARLY: COMPLICATIONS

When people are diagnosed with diabetes, their greatest fear is often about having to live a compromised life. My greatest fear is that they won't take care of themselves and will have to deal with diabetic complications. I don't like to talk about this aspect of the disease. But any discussion of diabetes requires a reality check about its potential complications. If high blood sugar levels didn't harm us, we wouldn't care about them. But high blood sugar levels, over time, can—and do—cause disastrous problems. So I am compelled to define the nature of these complications—not to scare you, but to make you aware of how serious they are.

If high blood sugar levels didn't harm us,
we wouldn't care about them.

Every day in my practice I see many healthy patients with diabetes. I see patients who lead active, fulfilling lives, and who are unlikely to ever develop significant diabetic complications. I have patients who have lived with diabetes for more than fifty years and are still going strong: golfing, playing tennis, traveling, eating out in fine restaurants, enjoying marriage—in other words, simply aging normally.

So much of diabetes is about helping yourself.

Seeing these individuals makes me tremendously happy, because I also see the darker side of the story. At least once a week, if not once a day, I see a patient who has not had good diabetic control, and who must live with terrible complications. I see patients in their twenties and thirties who are going blind or going on dialysis or who have lost parts of their feet and legs. I have seen people in their thirties and forties die from overwhelming complications of diabetes. Poorly treated diabetes is like cancer and can be equally devastating and just as rapid. When I see these patients decline, I wish I could have seen them sooner. So much of diabetes is about helping yourself. That's why I stress to everyone with diabetes just how preventable these awful complications are, and what can be done to avoid them.

In general, there are two types of diabetes complications: the microvascular (small blood vessel) complications and the macrovascular (large blood vessel) complications. The microvascular complications are the ones that involve the eyes, the kidneys, and the nerves. The macrovascular complications are those that involve the larger blood vessels, and include coronary artery disease, stroke, peripheral vascular disease, and heart attack. There is a different approach used for preventing each set of complications, although often strategies to avoid the microvascular complications will help the macrovascular complications and vice versa.

Microvascular Complications (Eyes, Kidneys, Nerves)

The microvascular complications appear to be almost entirely caused by high levels of blood sugar. It is not known exactly how high blood sugars cause these complications. It is clear, though, that high sugar levels cause damage to the fragile lining of blood vessels and other tissues that eventually can result in their malfunction. Study after study has shown that the single best way to reduce the risk of, or avoid completely, the microvascular complications of diabetes is to maintain blood glucose levels as close to normal as possible.

Diabetic retinopathy is damage to the back of the eye (the retina), which is where the biomechanics of vision occur. The blood vessels in the back of the eye are extremely sensitive to the effects of glucose. In ways we do not quite understand, high levels of glucose make these blood vessels leak fluid—blood and other substances—into the back of the eye. When this happens, the delicate nerve cells that are involved in the transmission of vision can be damaged and, ultimately, destroyed. The amazing thing about diabetic retinopathy is that you can have terrible damage to the back of the eye, but if it does not involve the center of vision there may be no noticeable visual loss. But if not tracked carefully, vision may be adversely affected and it may be too late to do much about it. This is why the American Diabetes Association and I strongly recommend going to an eye doctor for a dilated eye examination at least once a year. That way, early, asymptomatic changes to the back of the eye can be detected and treated before retinopathy can progress from visual impairment to blindness.

Kidney damage is equally insidious. Patients with diabetes often have no idea they have any damage to their kidneys until their kidneys are seriously injured. Fortunately, there usually is an early warning signal in the form of leakage of small amounts of protein into the urine. If such leakage is detected, there are medications that can be used to help prevent kidneys from eventually failing. Therefore, patients with diabetes should have a urine test for microalbuminuria done every year; this reliable test measures protein *in relation to* another substance, creatinine. Surprisingly, many physicians do not consider this test necessary, although many medical associations recommend it for patients with diabetes. Most general doctors tend to do what is called simply a urine test for protein; this test detects only the presence of protein. Protein, however, is a later sign of kidney damage, and it is crucial to pick up any signs of kidney damage as early as possible; the microalbuminuria test is always quicker to show a problem.

The American Diabetes Association and I strongly recommend going to an eye doctor for a dilated eye examination at least once a year.

Diabetic neuropathy, or damage to the nerves, is a process that unfortunately gives no early warning signs. The most prevalent form of diabetic neuropathy involves numbness, tingling, or pain in the feet. Diabetic nerve damage, at least this common sort, tends to be in both feet. There are many other forms of diabetic neuropathy affecting the function of individual groups of nerves in other parts of the body. Once these neuropathic events occur, they either resolve by themselves or are treated with pain medications. Neuropathy generally comes on ten to twenty years after the diagnosis of diabetes. As with other forms of complications, the best way to prevent neuropathy is to control blood sugar levels. Many researchers are working on ways to help reverse and/or more effectively treat neuropathy but, thus far, the best approach clearly is prevention.

Macrovascular Complications
(Heart Attack, Stroke, Peripheral Vascular Disease)

Everyone who has prediabetes or diabetes is at risk for having heart disease, which affects the body's large blood vessels. Problems with the large blood vessels can cause a heart attack or, sometimes, a stroke. You must therefore do whatever possible to lower your heart attack potential. I used to think that treating diabetes was just about lowering blood sugar, but now I know that it is just as much about lowering cholesterol, triglyceride, and blood pressure levels, too. Rarely do I treat a patient with type 2 diabetes with just medication to lower blood sugar levels. As I'll explain later (chapter 13), treating type 2 diabetes means also using many different treatments to lower the risk for macrovascular disease. I also prescribe other medications for my type 1 patients to help prevent macrovascular problems.

I used to think that treating diabetes was just about lowering blood sugar, but now I know that it is just as much about lowering cholesterol, triglyceride, and blood pressure levels, too.

Macrovascular complications involve clogged blood vessels. When the blood vessels to your heart become clogged, you have a heart attack. If the blood vessels to the brain get clogged, you can have a stroke. Other blood vessels, such as the ones to the legs, can get clogged as well, leading to pain and sometimes amputation of the toes, foot, or leg. The risk for these complications can be diminished by taking medication to lower cholesterol levels, by keeping blood pressure in the normal range, and by lessening the risk of clot formation (which is usually accomplished by taking aspirin). Keeping blood sugars near normal also probably helps reduce the chance of macrovascular complications, but the impact is less clear than it is with microvascular complications.

TABLE 3. COMPLICATIONS FROM DIABETES: TESTS AND TREATMENTS

Complication	Test for Early Detection	Treatment
Eye damage	Dilated eye exam	Laser therapy
Kidney damage	Urine measurement of A/C ratio*	ACE inhibitors and/or ARBs[†]
Nerve damage	Symptoms of tingling or pain in your feet	None except to keep blood sugar normal and take pain medication
Foot ulcers and amputations	Check your feet every day	Early ulcers can be treated by a podiatrist before they spread
Risk for heart attack and stroke	Measure cholesterol and triglyceride levels and blood pressure	Treat cholesterol with drugs and keep blood pressure less than 130/80 mmHg; take aspirin daily

*See pages 151–152.
†See page 136.

STARTING THE JOURNEY TO HEALTH

Again, I apologize for having to talk about the frightening downside of diabetes. Please remember that complications are mostly preventable with good blood sugar control and are not inevitable outcomes of a diabetes diagnosis. No matter whether you have prediabetes, type 1, or type 2, the focus of your treatment is on reducing the risks of, and preventing, complications. With the right medication and some effort on your part, I know that you can live a long and healthy life with diabetes. And that life begins with knowing not only the right questions to ask, but who to ask and when to ask them.

Please remember that complications are mostly preventable with good blood sugar control and are not inevitable outcomes of a diabetes diagnosis.

THREE

THE BEST POSSIBLE HEALTH CARE BEGINS WITH YOU

Diabetes is subtle. It is not like having a heart attack. What often happens with patients is that they say, "Yes, I have diabetes. Now I'll let my doctor take care of it." If you do that, odds are that you won't receive adequate care and you will put yourself at great risk for complications. In order to stay well, you have to learn how to navigate your own health care situation and take control of your health.

In many cases just following up with your physician isn't good enough. Much of the information on prediabetes is so new that many doctors aren't aware of what they can do to treat it. Patients with diabetes often receive less than optimal diabetes care, both because it is complex and time-consuming and because the goals are hard to achieve. I want you to understand the way diabetes works. With this disease, what the patient does is as important as the doctor's prescribed treatment. Staying healthy with prediabetes and diabetes is within your power. You just have to know how to effectively locate, assemble, and use the health care resources available to you.

HOW TO FIND GOOD HEALTH CARE

No matter what health care system you have access to, you can find a way to get good care for prediabetes and diabetes. I run a diabetes center for poor, uninsured people in Los Angeles and know that even people with limited access to health care can still find health care providers and centers where controlling their diabetes is possible. The necessary elements for getting good care include being knowledgeable about your disease and taking advantage of the monitoring and treatments that are available. You must learn the questions to ask and be brave enough to question your health care providers until you find the answers you need.

When I give talks to doctors about preventing diabetes, I am always shocked at how many come up to me afterward worried about *themselves*. Many are at high risk but have done nothing about it until they hear me speak. This is either because they didn't even know they were at risk in the first place or, if they knew their risk, they didn't know exactly what to do about it. If a doctor isn't able to recognize this risk in himself, what is the likelihood that he will recognize it in you? I want to help you to become enough of an expert yourself to know to go to your doctor and ask about your risk for diabetes. I want you to be able to understand if you are getting the correct and complete answers. And, if not, I want you to know what to do next.

When I give talks to doctors about preventing diabetes, I am always shocked at how many come up to me afterward worried about themselves.

It is not sufficient to passively accept the health care you are offered. You don't do this when you are buying a car. When you buy a car you shop around, test-drive various models, compare the options, and finally settle on the car that is best for you. The same should be true for health care—we medical people are the providers, you are the consumer. However, unlike car shopping, where more money will buy you a fancier model, in medicine things work differently. Doctors are basically paid the same whether they do a good or a bad job. So it is up to you to discern whether you are getting the quality of health care you want. If not, you can either change your health care providers and/or change your insurance plan until you find the care you are looking for.

My patient Ruth Netter is a great example of how persistence in finding good health care has led to lifelong good health. She's an eighty-three-year-old widow who has had type 2 diabetes since 1960. She leads a very active life and, other than a small heart attack a few years ago, she has experienced no diabetes complications. And, although she complains about her doctors (because she doesn't like to be told to lose weight), in every city she's lived in she has tried to find the best medical care possible and has worked to treat her diabetes as well as she could.

....

"Diabetes is in my genes."

Diabetes is in my genes. My maternal grandmother, Bubbie Chana, was one of the first to benefit from the discovery of insulin. She lived in

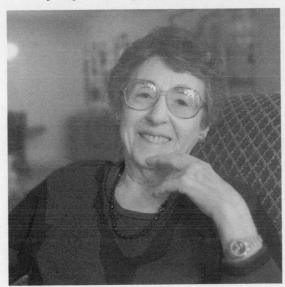

Toronto when Dr. Banting discovered this new "wonder drug." As a child I remember my grandmother giving us the little wooden boxes with the sliding lids, which protected her vials of insulin. She lived to the age of eighty-two.

When my parents were in their forties they both developed type 2 diabetes. So it was not a big surprise when, at the age of thirty-nine while in preparation for surgery, I was found to have diabetes. (Back then we didn't know what prediabetes was.) My internist put me on oral meds, cautioned me to avoid anything with sugar, and told me to "lose weight." Since I had been battling the bulge all my life, I guess my attitude was "so what's new?" I was not much good at following his advice.

Over the years we moved around the country. With each move I tried to find the best possible health care, either through recommendations from friends who were in health care or through the universities where my husband worked. Although I was frustrated by being told to "lose weight" without any specific recommendations about how to do it,

I was able to keep my diabetes under control with oral medications, exercise, and an awareness of the need to eat a healthy diet.

My husband retired in 1983 and we moved back to Los Angeles. I found an endocrinologist recommended by a friend, who was a nurse. Did this new doctor tell me to lose weight? Of course—and once again I lost a little, but once again it was not enough. During one visit he asked if I would like to participate in a study for a drug called metformin, to be conducted by Dr. Anne Peters. By joining this study I was put in touch with the newest ways to treat diabetes. I benefited personally, not only from the study medication but from the team of health care providers who were available to help me. They helped me understand that the success or failure of my care did not depend on the seemingly impossible goal of losing weight. They also helped put that goal in perspective with all of the other goals of my care. With a new attitude and a revised approach, I was able to control my diabetes well and even lose weight. I have stayed with this team of health care providers ever since. I am now eighty-three years old. I live alone, volunteer in my community, and feel great most of the time.

I have two suggestions for living a long and healthy life with diabetes. First, read nutrition labels on everything you are thinking of purchasing. When I do this I put back as many items as I buy. Being aware of the calories, sugar, fat, and carbohydrate count has helped me lose weight—at long last! Second, the most important thing you can do is to find a health care team who takes care of your diabetes and cares about you as a person. The partnership you form can help you for many years to come.

....

PUTTING TOGETHER YOUR TEAM FOR A HEALTHY LIFE

How can you be as successful as Ruth and live a "long and healthy life" with diabetes? The first person you are likely to look to is your regular doctor, the one you are used to seeing. You depend on your physician to give you a complete evaluation, diagnosis, and treatment plan. But what happens if your doctor doesn't know much about diabetes or doesn't have enough time to spend with you? A routine medical visit usually lasts between seven and twelve minutes. This is generally enough time to measure your blood pressure and your weight, ask how you are feeling, examine some limited part of you, give you a prescription or two, and tell you when to return. If you happen to have an acute problem, such as an earache or a painful knee, that issue will consume all of the time your doctor has to spend with you.

A routine medical visit usually lasts between seven and twelve minutes.

This lack of time is not necessarily your physician's fault. As technology and medication costs increase, payments to physicians decrease; they can afford to spend less and less time with each patient. I was consulting at one medical group where the director shared with me that his goal was to limit each physician visit to a three-minute encounter. Three minutes! How can quality care be provided in so short a time? It can't. Additionally, this medical director (and many others I have spoken to) doesn't care much about preventing chronic complications because one-quarter of the patients leave his group's health plan each year. So by the time someone needs expensive care, such as laser eye surgery or heart bypass surgery, someone else will foot the bill.

These are grim realities, and undoubtedly you are aware of them. But you can do something about it because, to a large extent, you are responsible for your own health care. That doesn't mean you have to go it alone. In fact, I think every patient should have a group of health care providers to work with. In other words, a team.

A SAMPLE HEALTH CARE TEAM

1. A compassionate *primary care physician* who listens to your questions and understands diabetes.

2. An *endocrinologist* if you take insulin, or feel that your prediabetes or diabetes is not being well treated.

3. A *diabetes educator/nurse* and/or a *nutritionist* with a special interest in diabetes who can spend the time with you to teach

you what you need to know to best manage the disease. Often these individuals are CDEs (certified diabetes educators).

4. An *ophthalmologist* (eye doctor) to see at least once a year who is an expert in diabetic eye disease.

5. A *podiatrist* (foot doctor) with an interest in diabetes if you have neuropathy (numb or painful feet) or a history of foot ulcers.

How to Choose Your Physician

When you are shopping (yes, *shopping*) for health care, it is perfectly acceptable to tell a physician you are meeting for the first time that you are in the process of interviewing doctors to find the setting that suits you best. For example, patients with special-needs adult children have had screening visits with me and have asked me for second opinions, which I am always happy to give. It is very important to me that patients find a doctor who fills their expectations—even if it isn't me.

I often will ask a new patient what they didn't like about their prior health care provider. This allows me to come up with strategies to satisfy the patient's needs. Sometimes this is as simple as telling a patient what to expect from me—when I will report back on lab tests, how often patients should come to the clinic, how to reach me (phone, e-mail, and pager) if a problem or question occurs. If your physician doesn't offer a plan for ongoing contact, you should ask when and how you should expect to hear about your lab and test results and how to reach your physician in case of an emergency.

I frequently see patients who have been with one doctor for many years and are afraid of "hurting his feelings" by seeking a second opinion or seeing a new doctor. This shouldn't be about any one physician's feelings; it is about what is best for *you*. And although sometimes I am sad when a patient chooses to see another physician instead of me, what I want in my heart is the best care for each person. So don't worry about disappointing your doctor; the most important issue is that you find health care providers you like and trust.

When looking for a doctor, you want someone who will listen to you and take the time to answer your questions. Even the best doctors don't know everything. In my opinion, one of the key features to being a truly great doctor is knowing when to ask for another opinion. Your physician (or her backup) should be available in case of emergency. Your doctor should never make you feel guilty for not "complying" with what she tells you to do. The word "failure" should never be part of a medical visit, and yet patients tell me all the time that they feel like failures.

Even the best doctors don't know everything.

It is important that your physician encourages you to try to get better and believes in your ability to become healthier, or to maintain your health if your health is good. Your physician should be helpful in referring you to see other providers, if you need additional help. Telling you to "go and lose weight" or to "start exercising" without providing you with specific advice and someone to help you make these changes is simply not enough. Nor is giving you a preprinted piece of paper with diet instructions on it. You are an individual and deserve individual help and guidance as you deal with prediabetes and diabetes.

When to See an Endocrinologist

As I discussed earlier, many people will not be able to see an endocrinologist who specializes in the treatment of prediabetes and diabetes. I spend a lot of time trying to teach primary care doctors how to treat diabetes. In the rest of this book I am going to teach you pretty much the same thing, so you'll know how to help yourself. Still, if you have type 1 diabetes or have difficult-to-control type 2 diabetes, it really helps to have an endocrinologist involved in your care. If you live far away from a big city with an endocrinologist you like, you can still arrange to fly in for an initial visit and then return twice a year for follow-up. In between, you can e-mail or fax in your blood sugar values. I do this for patients all over the country. Occasionally, I have people fly in from as far away as Miami or New York to see me, and I routinely see patients from around the state of California. As long as you have a good general doctor nearby who can take care of your basic medical needs and treat any emergencies that come up, I (or another endocrinologist) can help manage your diabetes care from afar. If you don't have or can't find a local diabetes specialist, then by all means look beyond your community for the care you need. The Internet can be a helpful tool in this research.

The Vital Role of Diabetes Educators and Nutritionists

I'm a big believer in the team approach to health care. Just as in team sports no one player can do it all, in diabetes management no one person can provide all the answers and all the help you need. In addition to a doctor or endocrinologist, you'll want a few other "players" and "coaches" on your health care team.

A good nurse educator or nutritionist may be able to teach you far more about day-to-day living with your diabetes than a physician can.

If at all possible you should find a nutritionist who is expert in the treatment of diabetes. You'll also want a good diabetes educator on your team. A diabetes educator, often a nurse, can teach you about monitoring your blood sugar levels, giving yourself injections (if necessary), and the best ways for you and your family to live with your diabetes. You may also want to attend diabetes classes, which are held at many local hospitals. At these classes you will not only learn about diabetes, you will meet other people who are in the same situation as you are.

A good nurse educator or nutritionist may be able to teach you far more about day-to-day living with your diabetes than a physician can. In your search for good medical care, you should look for professionals who are certified diabetes educators (CDEs). A CDE can be a nurse or a nutritionist or even a physician. It means that the provider has a special interest in giving diabetes education. If you can find a nurse or dietitian who is a CDE in your community he or she can be a great source for answers to your questions. Sometimes you may find one before you find a doctor, in which case the CDE may also be able to recommend a physician who is particularly good at treating patients with diabetes. Some communities have American Diabetes Association (ADA)–recognized diabetes programs; to obtain this recognition, the program must have a team of diabetes health care providers. You can look at the ADA website (www.diabetes.org), or call the ADA (1-800-342-2383) to find a list of recognized programs in your area.

Ophthalmologists and Podiatrists

Other team members can be backups, providers you only see annually, irregularly, or if special situations or problems develop. For example, you will need to have an eye doctor (ophthalmologist) for an annual dilated eye exam. You also may need to see a podiatrist (a foot doctor). Other potential team members include a cardiologist (heart doctor), nephrologist (kidney doctor), and therapist. Some people have a team of just one or two people and others have much larger diabetes teams. But what matters most is that you have providers you trust, you understand, and who seem to be able and willing to guide you as you learn to live with diabetes.

FIVE HEALTH CARE TEAMWORK TIPS

1. Assemble a health care team that partners with you in treating your diabetes. Team members should include a primary care doctor (who could be an endocrinologist), a nutritionist and/or a diabetes educator, an eye doctor, and possibly a foot doctor.

2. Communicate with your team regularly. Be sure you know how to reach your physician in an emergency.

3. Work with your team to tailor your treatment to your lifestyle.

4. Ask questions at every visit. Bring notes, questions, articles, and anything else that helps you remember what you want to learn more about.

5. Become your own expert. Read and learn as much as you can so you're always one step ahead in your prediabetes and diabetes care. *You* are the leader of the team.

PREPARING FOR YOUR VISITS

Whether you are going to see your primary care physician, your endocrinologist, or your diabetes educator, you should prepare for your visit. I always encourage patients to bring a list of questions with them so I am certain to address all of their concerns. I will often take the list from a patient and answer each question, writing down what I think is important as an answer. Patients also write down the answers themselves. It's hard to remember all that you hear in a medical visit so writing down the information can help you recall what's important later on. You should also bring articles or books or anything else that you want to share. Sometimes patients bring me articles about studies I haven't read about yet. (Medical news occasionally is published in the *Los Angeles Times* before it shows up in medical journals.) This motivates me to keep current and to find and read the original studies. Other times I can help patients interpret what they read in the media— often stories about medicine aren't accurate or they sensationalize experiments on mice or rats that are far from being applicable to human beings.

I also ask patients under treatment by other doctors to bring me any lab results, radiology reports, hospitalization summaries— whatever they have—so I can review and keep copies with their charts. That way, I don't unnecessarily repeat tests and will understand what is happening with their other health issues. You should keep copies of all of your medical records for your files, as noted below.

Important Medical Records

1. *All of your doctor's chart notes.* These are the notes he or she keeps from each visit. It helps to have the initial notes, which are usually the longest, and those from the most recent follow-up visits.

2. *Information concerning all hospitalizations.* This doesn't mean every page. As physicians we write admission notes (which describe why you came to the hospital) and discharge notes

(which describe what happened while you were there).
Usually, having these two summaries is adequate; if more
information is needed, your doctor can order it from the
hospital.

3. *A copy of your laboratory data.* Sometimes this comes conve-
niently organized on one flow sheet; other times it adds up
to many separate pages.

4. *A copy of all major test results.* These may include an X-ray,
MRI, CAT scan, ultrasound, biopsy, treadmill test, cardiac
echo, EKG, and pathology reports. Unless you have a very
unusual condition, usually a copy of the printed reports
from these tests is enough. Sometimes your doctor will need
a copy of the actual images (such as the X-ray or MRI) but
you will be asked for this either before your first visit or
shortly afterward.

Organize the information chronologically. I, for one, spend quite
a bit of time flipping through disorganized medical records trying
to make sense of them.

YOUR MEDICAL RECORDS: AN IMPORTANT TOOL
IN TREATING YOUR PREDIABETES AND DIABETES

You must always remember that your medical records are just
that—*your* medical records—contrary to how office staff may sometimes treat them. You should ask to have a copy of all actual blood
test results, as well as a copy of results of all tests that have been performed (such as X-rays, CAT scans, MRIs, surgical procedures, Pap
smears). If you do not understand a test result, you should ask what
it means. Some physicians say they don't want to give patients their
actual results because the patients won't understand what they
mean. It is true that you won't have the perspective a physician
would. We are taught to look for patterns of abnormalities, and
certain small changes in laboratory values may mean something serious to us. Sometimes, though, you can do as well as or even better than your physician. For instance, if you have prediabetes and
notice that your fasting blood sugar level has increased from 102

mg/dl one year to 110 mg/dl the next this could be a sign that you are moving closer to having diabetes and you may need to change your treatment. You should follow your laboratory results over time and consult your health care provider if you see them changing.

**Sometimes, though, you can do as well as
or even better than your physician.**

What I do with patients is go over their lab sheets with them and discuss every abnormality—explaining what it is about each that is important or not and why. You may need to make several appointments to have all your initial questions answered. This could get expensive and time-consuming, but you may feel it's necessary. Even if your physician tells you to come back in three months it is okay if you schedule an appointment sooner so you can ask all of your questions. Do not, however, expect your physician to spend much time speaking with you on the phone—phone calls should generally be used for true emergencies or for providing requested information (such as blood sugar levels after a medication change). Physicians, unlike attorneys, don't receive reimbursement for time spent on the phone and it can be very difficult to squeeze in phone calls during a busy day in a clinic. The exception to this is some diabetes educators, often nurses or dietitians, who will have time for telephone follow-up. You clearly should take advantage of this service if it is available.

PART TWO

PREVENTING DIABETES

THE HIDDEN DISORDERS: SYNDROME X, THE METABOLIC SYNDROME, INSULIN RESISTANCE SYNDROME, AND PREDIABETES

I am thrilled when patients arrive for their appointments armed with the kinds of questions that make me proud that I do what I do. I'm especially happy when new patients ask, "Am I at risk for getting diabetes? And, if so, how can I prevent it from developing?" In the past, most patients who came to see me were ill with diabetes, some with complications, others trying to prevent them, but all dealing with a high blood sugar level and its effects on their bodies. Now, due to increased awareness, people who have a friend or family member with diabetes or who have read about the risk factors for prediabetes are taking the initiative and coming to my center, where we screen for prediabetes and diabetes.

Screening also can be done by your primary care physician, but because diabetes is something I specialize in, I do tests that are above and beyond the basic. Then, I take the time to teach patients what their test results mean—for the present and in the future. I am also more prone to use diabetes medications to treat prediabetes before such drugs are approved for general diabetes prevention. As I explain below, I use data from the latest studies to give recommendations prior to changes in FDA guidelines. Because I have so much experience in using these medications, and particularly because of my access to the most recent research, I am comfortable in treating patients more aggressively than a general physician might be. It is so much better to see a patient before he has a heart attack or gets diabetes, or before diabetic complications set in. Of course, the preventive visits are not quite as dramatic as the ones where big, life-changing treatment changes are made. In the preventive visits I deal with small changes in blood sugars, blood cholesterol, and blood pressure. From everything we know, though, these seemingly small changes can make a lasting difference for years to come.

PREDIABETES BY ANY OTHER NAME

"Syndrome X"—the name for the time before you get diabetes, when you have insulin resistance but not high blood sugar levels— was coined by Dr. Gerald Reaven, a very well known diabetes researcher at Stanford (who helped me when I did my training there) and one of the first people to talk about the condition. Unfortunately, this term already had been used for an obscure heart ailment. So the official name was changed to "insulin resistance syndrome." Cardiologists (heart specialists, who are very interested in this phase of illness since it so often leads to heart disease) wanted to call it the "metabolic syndrome." The American Diabetes Association (more focused on glucose) wants it called "prediabetes."

The bottom line is that it doesn't matter what you call it. What matters is that you are alert to the fact that it can exist so you can take action to find medical care for it. For the purposes of this book I am going to call it "prediabetes" because that is the simplest to remember and links it to the progression to diabetes. Insulin resistance and the metabolic syndrome are the broader problems. Because we don't have specific clinical tests to determine whether insulin resistance is present or not, it is harder to define and talk about. We can do advanced tests in the laboratory to measure what is going on in someone's body, but not in nonresearch subjects.

The bottom line is that it doesn't matter what you call it.

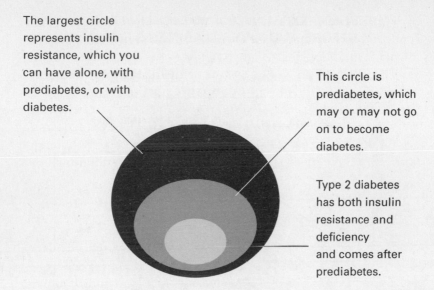

The largest circle represents insulin resistance, which you can have alone, with prediabetes, or with diabetes.

This circle is prediabetes, which may or may not go on to become diabetes.

Type 2 diabetes has both insulin resistance and deficiency and comes after prediabetes.

The diagram above shows how insulin resistance, prediabetes, and diabetes are interrelated. The circles correspond to how many people have each condition: more have insulin resistance alone than have prediabetes; more have prediabetes than diabetes. Everyone with insulin resistance, or at least most of them, pose a risk for a heart attack. People with type 2 diabetes (insulin resistance plus insulin deficiency) have additional risks for the complications of diabetes, including blindness, kidney failure, and amputation.

INSULIN RESISTANCE: A KEY CONCEPT IN DIABETES PREVENTION

Insulin resistance starts long before you develop diabetes—often fifteen to twenty years before blood sugar levels begin to increase. Insulin resistance means that your body doesn't respond normally to the insulin it makes. Several things cause insulin resistance—for example, simply getting older makes all of us more insulin resistant. But if you are overweight, don't exercise much, or have a family history of diabetes you are at increased risk for having insulin resistance. Insulin resistance makes your pancreas work extra hard to make enough insulin to keep your blood sugar levels normal.

INSULIN RESISTANCE AND INSULIN LEVELS
BEFORE AND AFTER DIABETES STARTS

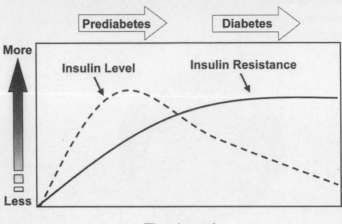

Time (years)

Over time, your pancreas "burns out" and you can't make enough insulin to keep your blood sugar levels down. The resulting insulin deficiency happens gradually, and your blood sugar levels rise slowly. By the time diabetes develops you have both insulin resistance and insulin deficiency.

Look at the chart above. I want to use it to make a few very important points. First, it shows that you can have a *normal* blood sugar level (below 100 mg/dl) for years before any increase is seen. During this period of escalating insulin resistance, even though blood sugar levels are normal you are still at increased risk for heart disease. There is no official name for this period of time *before* prediabetes and diabetes (since both prediabetes and diabetes are diagnosed based on blood sugar levels only). As I mentioned before, some people call it the "metabolic syndrome" and others call it by the more mysterious-sounding "syndrome X." The risk factors for it are the same as for prediabetes and type 2 diabetes; it is just an earlier part of the same process.

The way you know that you have insulin resistance involves the same indicators as prediabetes. If you are overweight (especially around the middle), have abnormal lipids (high triglyceride levels and low levels of HDL, or good cholesterol) and high blood pressure, you are almost certain to have insulin resistance—even with a normal fasting blood sugar level. The treatments for insulin resistance and prediabetes are identical—both are designed to lower your risk for diabetes and heart disease, so I use the terms interchangeably.

Insulin resistance not only makes your body less sensitive to insulin, it also seems to cause an increase in the risk for heart attack and stroke. There have been many studies of the risk of heart attack conducted by investigators from all over the world, such as Bo Isomaa and colleagues in Finland and Sweden, Steven Haffner and his group in San Antonio, and Frank Hu at Harvard.[1] These studies have found that for as long as fifteen years before the actual onset of diabetes there is double the risk of heart attack compared to people without insulin resistance. Put another way, when we diagnose someone with "new" type 2 diabetes, half of those people will already have heart disease. Clearly, we need to do something sooner, long before someone develops diabetes, so we can prevent the beginnings of complications.

TESTING FOR INSULIN RESISTANCE

There are six basic factors that can indicate if you are at risk for having insulin resistance:

1. Being overweight (body mass index of 25 or greater)

2. Too little HDL (good) cholesterol (less than 40 mg/dl if male; less than 50 if female)

3. A triglyceride level that is too high (above 150 mg/dl)

4. High blood pressure (above 130/80 mmHg)

5. Elevated fasting blood sugar level (above 100 mg/dl)

6. Protein in your urine

The more of these abnormalities that you have, the more likely you are to have insulin resistance and prediabetes. Except for being overweight, I think all of these require a health care provider to determine. Your risk for insulin resistance also is increased if you have a history of diabetes in your family, which we've covered previously.

How to Calculate Your Body Mass Index (BMI)

Being overweight is the strongest risk factor for having insulin resistance and prediabetes. Although most of us know when we weigh more than we should, the medical field likes specific numbers. What we want to know is what your weight is relative to your height because this allows us to compare people of varying heights and weights with one another. If you try to imagine a person who is 6 feet tall and weighs 175 pounds you will think of someone who has a good body weight to height ratio. Now imagine the same person, weighing the same 175 pounds, but a foot shorter. The image of this five-foot-tall, 175-pound person is a lot different—akin to comparing a bowling pin to a bowling ball. In order to talk about this height and weight relationship we use the term "body mass index" (BMI). The calculation for figuring out BMI is body weight (in kilograms) divided by height (in meters) squared (kg/m2). An easy way to determine your BMI is to find your weight and height on a table (below) or to do the calculation on a special Internet site (http://nhlbisupport.com/bmi/bmicalc.htm).

What we want to know is what your weight is relative to your height because this allows us to compare people of varying heights and weights with one another.

You want to have a BMI of less than 25. Average people, ones whom you would look at and say, "That person looks good" probably have a BMI of 20 to 23. Most skinny fashion models have a BMI of 17 or 18. If your BMI is greater than 25 you are considered overweight, and greater than 30 is very overweight or obese.

Are You an Apple or a Pear?

I have long used Homer Simpson as my "poster boy" for prediabetes and insulin resistance. He is drawn to show someone who is

TABLE 4. BODY MASS INDEX

BMI	19	20	21	22	23	24	25	26	27	28	29	30	31	32	33	34	35	36	37
Height	Normal						Overweight					Obese							
4' 10"	91	96	100	105	110	115	119	124	129	134	139	143	148	153	158	163	167	173	177
4' 11"	94	99	104	109	114	119	124	128	133	138	143	148	153	158	163	169	173	179	183
5' 0"	97	102	107	113	118	123	128	133	138	143	148	153	159	164	169	175	179	185	189
5' 1"	100	106	111	116	122	127	132	137	143	148	153	158	164	169	174	180	185	191	196
5' 2"	104	109	115	120	126	131	136	142	147	153	158	164	169	175	180	186	191	197	202
5' 3"	107	113	118	124	130	135	141	146	152	158	164	169	175	181	187	192	198	204	209
5' 4"	110	116	122	128	134	140	145	151	157	163	169	174	180	187	193	199	204	210	215
5' 5"	114	120	126	132	138	144	150	156	162	168	174	180	186	193	199	205	210	217	222
5' 6"	118	124	130	136	142	148	155	161	167	173	179	186	192	199	205	211	217	224	229
5' 7"	121	127	134	140	147	153	159	166	172	178	185	191	198	205	212	218	224	230	236
5' 8"	125	131	138	145	151	158	164	171	177	184	191	197	204	211	218	224	230	237	243
5' 9"	128	135	142	149	156	162	169	176	182	189	196	203	210	217	223	231	237	244	250
5' 10"	132	139	146	153	160	167	174	181	188	195	202	207	216	223	230	237	244	251	258
5' 11"	136	143	150	158	165	172	179	186	193	200	208	215	222	230	236	244	251	259	265
6' 0"	140	147	154	162	269	177	184	191	199	206	214	221	228	236	243	251	258	266	273
6' 1"	144	151	159	167	174	182	189	197	204	212	220	227	235	243	250	258	265	273	280
6' 2"	148	155	163	171	179	187	194	202	210	218	226	233	241	250	257	265	272	281	288
6' 3"	152	160	168	176	184	192	200	208	216	224	232	240	248	256	264	272	280	289	297
6' 4"	156	164	172	181	189	197	205	213	222	230	238	246	254	263	271	280	288	296	304

Weight (pounds)

overweight, but very specifically someone who is overweight in the middle—the classic "apple" or "O" shape. I am not sure whether or not artist Matt Groening knew he was drawing a prototype for prediabetes, but if you look like Homer—and have his unhealthy eating and exercise (that is, none) habits—you are at risk.

I am not the only one who has noted this association. I remember hearing a radio report on some scientists in Great Britain who decided to determine how fat Homer is based on what he looks like on television. They concluded that he has an unhealthy BMI of 34.

If you look like Homer—and have his unhealthy eating and exercise (that is, none) habits—you are at risk.

Homer also is an illustration of the fact that not all fat bodies are the same. Much of his fat is around his middle. This body shape is said to have "central obesity," with relatively thin legs and arms. Other people gain fat all over, with an excess in the buttocks, hips, and thighs (the "pear" or "A" shape). The apple shape is the one that is most commonly seen in patients with insulin resistance and diabetes. The apple shape (central obesity) is the most dangerous and puts people at highest risk for developing heart disease and diabetes. Pear people are at less risk.

Recently it has been learned that fat cells are capable of making and releasing hormones that have many different effects on the body. Some of these hormones make us feel hungry; others make us feel full. Still others cause insulin resistance and some make us more insulin sensitive. The worst type of fat seems to be the central or visceral fat deposited around the middle. If you were to look inside a person with a big belly you would see lots of white fat draped around their liver, pancreas, and intestines. Such inner fat causes all sorts of problems for those internal organs, making it harder for them to work and causing insulin resistance and diabetes.

The worst type of fat seems to be the central or visceral fat deposited around the middle.

As bad as this sounds (and as dangerous as it is), it is a wonderful adaptation for survival. As I mentioned in the first chapter, this kind of central, internal fat once worked as a great storage place for nutrients that helped humans survive periods of starvation. When our ancient ancestors couldn't find food, they lived off their internal fat, sometimes for extended periods. (Remember the "thrifty genes"?) Now that our food supply is essentially secure, we don't have to worry as much about starvation. But the inner fat still builds up and, if not burned up through exercise, it releases dangerous substances into the bloodstream that cause inflammation, an irritation of the blood vessels, an increased risk for clotting, and abnormal cholesterol levels. This is why people with central fat are at such high risk for heart disease. These same toxins cause insulin resistance and, over time, also will cause insulin deficiency.

I usually don't measure someone's waist size. I just ask new patients where they gain weight and if they pat their center I assume they have a central pattern of weight gain. However, the official definition for central obesity is a waist circumference (measured around the middle, at the level of your belly button) of greater than 102 centimeters (40 inches) if you are male, and greater than 88 centimeters (35 inches) if you are female. This definition may not be applicable to all people. Asians, for example, tend to have smaller waist sizes for the same level of insulin resistance, and children's waist sizes change with growth.

Abnormal Cholesterol and Triglyceride Levels

One of the most important factors in insulin resistance (and, hence, in prediabetes and diabetes) is cholesterol level. Once or twice every month I see a patient who has just had a heart attack who wonders, "How could I have a heart attack? My doctor said I had a normal cholesterol level." Was the doctor wrong? No, the patient may well have had a normal level of total and low-density lipoprotein (LDL, or "bad") cholesterol. But what they also had was an abnormally low level of high-density lipoprotein (HDL, or "good") cholesterol that normally protects from LDL's adverse effects. There are many other abnormalities of blood vessels, inflammation, and coagulation caused by insulin resistance that lead to an increased risk of heart attack, but the one commonly measured marker that often is unaddressed is HDL cholesterol level.

This is broad and complex science, but in very simple terms heart attacks are almost always caused by a build-up of cholesterol on blood vessel walls. Deposits of cholesterol are also known as plaque. Abnormal fat and cholesterol levels in the blood can be readily measured by a fasting lipid panel. Your doctor should get four crucial numbers back relating your lipid levels. The first one is your total cholesterol level. This should be below 200 mg/dl. The next one is your triglyceride level. Increased triglyceride levels are a sign that you have insulin resistance. If they are above 150 mg/dl you are considered at risk. These high triglyceride levels indicate that your body isn't processing fat correctly, which often happens before your blood sugar levels go up noticeably. This also is why heart disease can happen before you get diabetes. When your triglyceride levels are high it makes your good (HDL) cholesterol levels fall, which in turn makes your bad (LDL) cholesterol particles smaller and denser. Think of it as a dangerous teeter-totter. High triglyceride levels themselves may not hurt you, but because they cause other problems they are evidence of a serious underlying disorder.

Increased triglyceride levels are a sign that you have insulin resistance.

After the total cholesterol and triglyceride levels, your lipid panel will give separate LDL (bad) and HDL (good) cholesterol levels. Your LDL level should be below 100 mg/dl (although recent research shows that an LDL below 70 mg/dl may be even better). And your HDL (good) cholesterol level needs to be above 40 mg/dl. If your HDL level drops below 40 if you are male, and 50 if you are female, it indicates a strong risk of insulin resistance and heart disease. Why? Because HDL cholesterol's job is to help remove bad cholesterol from your arteries. It functions sort of like a vacuum cleaner for cholesterol. If you have a lot of HDL cholesterol, it sucks up the cholesterol from your arteries and disposes of it in your liver (so it goes out into your gut).

There are two important things, then, you should ask your doctor about your lipid profile when it comes to prediabetes: (1) What is my triglyceride level? and (2) What is my HDL (good) cholesterol level? Usually, we just ask about total cholesterol, but these are different questions and are very important when it comes to assessing risk for heart disease and insulin resistance.

TABLE 5. TYPICAL LIPID PANEL RESULTS FROM SOMEONE WITH AND WITHOUT INSULIN RESISTANCE

Lipid Test	No Prediabetes	Prediabetes/Insulin Resistance
Total cholesterol level (the same)	174	174
Triglycerides	120	190
LDL (bad) cholesterol	90	106
HDL (good) cholesterol	60	30
Risk for heart attack	Low	High

Blood Pressure Basics

High blood pressure (hypertension) is a common problem, but it is much more prevalent in patients with prediabetes. If you test people with high blood pressure for insulin resistance, many of them will have it. There is not necessarily a concrete correlation between high blood pressure and increased risk for, or having, prediabetes. Likewise, low or normal blood pressure doesn't mean you won't have it. High blood pressure is just one of the possible indicators of prediabetes and should be treated as such. (Remember, we aren't diagnosing diabetes here, just a risk for developing it.) Many hormones are involved in the regulation of blood pressure. These can be at abnormal levels in patients with insulin resistance, resulting in high blood pressure (above 130/80 mmHg). When blood pressure is elevated, it causes extra stress on the heart as well as on the blood vessels that go to the brain and the kidneys. It is important for people with prediabetes and diabetes to keep blood pressure in the normal range because the heart and blood vessels already could be compromised.

When blood pressure is elevated, it causes extra stress on the heart as well as on the blood vessels that go to the brain and the kidneys.

When you have your blood pressure measured you should be sitting calmly on a chair. Your legs should not be crossed and your testing arm should be held at the level of your heart. You should make sure that the person testing your blood pressure uses the correct size blood pressure cuff. Blood pressure cuffs come in several sizes. A standard size works if you are not overweight. An adult large cuff can be used if you are overweight and an even larger cuff (a thigh cuff) can be used if you are quite large. If, on the other hand, you are quite small, you may need a child-sized cuff. The wrong size cuff can give an incorrect blood pressure reading; it obviously is important that you ask for a larger or smaller cuff if you are concerned about the fit. (You can gauge the fit yourself—the cuff shouldn't be straining around your arm; but should fit comfortably, closing easily in the center.)

There are two numbers associated with a blood pressure reading. Take as an example a blood pressure of 130/80 (spoken as "one thirty over eighty"). The first number (130) relates to "systolic" blood pressure (SBP) and is the number on the top. This is the higher number and corresponds to your heart pumping blood out. The lower number (80) is called the "diastolic" blood pressure (DBP) and relates to the pressure in your blood vessels when your heart muscle is between beats. The blood pressure is sort of the measurement of the ebb and flow of the beating of your heart. Think of the systolic blood pressure as the time of maximal force and the diastolic as the time of relaxation. Neither figure should be elevated because in either case it would indicate some problem in the regulation of force through your blood vessels which can damage them and cause heart attacks and strokes.

The blood pressure is sort of the measurement of the ebb and flow of the beating of your heart.

Many people come into my office with a high blood pressure reading and say that they have "white coat hypertension," or, in other words, a blood pressure level that increases when they see a doctor and get nervous. Regardless of the cause, it is still high blood pressure and can cause harm. It is likely that throughout any given day those same patients will encounter other stressful situations. A lower blood pressure is usually better, especially if you have prediabetes—unless it is so low that you feel dizzy or weak from any blood pressure medication you may be taking.

To help my patients get a sense of their blood pressure levels, I encourage them to buy a blood pressure cuff and check themselves at home. I usually have people test in the morning, just after they get up, and then later in the day. This gives both patient and doctor a sense of blood pressure over time, instead of on just one occasion in the doctor's office. You should ask your physician which blood pressure monitor he or she recommends and you may want to bring it into the office to test it against the blood pressure level measured there.

If prediabetes is picked up early and treated correctly, many of the complications, including the progression to diabetes, can be prevented.

Blood Sugar Level: The Final Sign

Ironically, the last sign of insulin resistance is an increase in fasting blood sugar levels. This is because the body can keep blood sugar levels in the normal range for a long time by making extra insulin.

Eventually, though, your body can't keep up with demand and your insulin secretion starts to fall. Blood sugar levels then start to rise.

If you were to measure your insulin levels when your blood sugar levels were normal (but with insulin resistance present) your fasting insulin levels would be increased. Unfortunately, measuring insulin levels accurately is difficult and so not recommended. If you can get your insulin level measured, and it is above 15, you have insulin resistance. Researchers are working to make better tests for measuring insulin levels; such tests may become commercially available in the next few years. In the laboratory in my clinic we can measure insulin levels reasonably well. I will order a test for it when a patient whom I think may have early insulin resistance has a blood sugar level that is below 100 mg/dl.

Most physicians now measure your fasting blood sugar level (after twelve hours without eating or drinking anything except for water). If your fasting blood sugar level is above 100, you have prediabetes. Rising "postprandial" (after eating) blood sugar levels will be the earliest signal, and sometimes doctors will perform an oral glucose tolerance test. It involves drinking a sugary sweet drink, usually disguised as a cola or orange drink; your blood sugar levels are checked before and then two hours after drinking it. As mentioned in chapter 1, this test is not recommended for general use since it takes two hours and the results can be quite variable. It may be done for research purposes or if a woman is being tested for diabetes during pregnancy. Sometimes doctors have a personal preference for this test, particularly if they have done a lot of research and want very specific answers. If your doctor recommends a glucose tolerance test you should ask why, and ask what additional information will be obtained that can't be learned from your fasting blood sugar level.

**If your fasting blood sugar level is above 100,
you have prediabetes.**

INSULIN RESISTANCE IS DANGEROUS BUT MANAGEABLE

Medical researchers don't yet understand all of the reasons why the four key elements of the prediabetes syndrome—obesity, abnormal cholesterol levels, high blood pressure, and elevated blood sugars—cause heart disease and diabetes. But their deadly relationship is well known. We think an interplay between genes and the environment leads to an increase in fat. The increase in fat and resulting lack of insulin sensitivity leads to abnormal lipids (cholesterol and triglycerides) in your blood, along with elevated blood pressure and blood sugar. Together, these are major factors in heart attacks and strokes. Other problems—which we usually don't measure, such as abnormal blood vessel functioning and an increase in inflammation and coagulation—also are present, increasing the risk for future diabetic complications.

If this syndrome goes on for long enough (and it often does, because it is not usually diagnosed early), it will turn into type 2 diabetes. Fortunately we know that if insulin resistance is picked up early and treated correctly, many of the complications, including the progression to diabetes, can be prevented. So don't despair. Once you are thinking about this problem, once you are reading this book and wondering what is going on with your body, you are already a big step ahead. With an awareness that you have prediabetes potential, you can do many things (including implement changes in lifestyle as well as begin medication) that can lower the risk back down toward normal.

....

"I didn't understand what was happening to me."

Lin Oliver's story points out the dangers of not diagnosing this syndrome and the questions we still have about what to do if you have it.

When I first saw the complications of insulin resistance I didn't know what it was. I found out many years later but by then it was too late to help my mother. She had developed symptoms of heart disease around the time my first son was born. She couldn't carry him across the room without clutching her chest in pain but she refused to undergo testing for her heart.

After my second son was born, however, she agreed to have a treadmill test. Within minutes of getting the results, she was taken for emergency bypass surgery. We were told that she had terrible blockages of her arteries, and that without surgery she would likely die within the year. She came out of the operating room late in the afternoon. All had gone well, she was fine, and we were sent home to rest. But at one AM she was rushed back to the operating room because she started to bleed uncontrollably from her heart.

In the days and months that followed, our sorrow and guilt were intense. But for me the concerns were even more personal. My mother and three of her nine siblings had died from heart disease. They all had hypertension, and several of them had diabetes. Our family was Jewish, from Hungary and Russia. All of us had apple shapes, with big stomachs and skinny legs. My mother, who did not have diabetes, was always slender, but she had the same build. All her weight was in the center. The thought of meeting the same fate as my mother terrified me.

I was soon pregnant with my third son. I had diet-controlled gestational diabetes with each of my two prior pregnancies, and my first two sons had each weighed more than nine pounds. With this third pregnancy, I was confined to bedrest, and had to take insulin injections to control my blood sugar levels. After my third son was born, I was told that I could develop diabetes in the future, but received no information on how to reduce this risk.

Eventually, when I went to see a new doctor, I was told that I needed a test for diabetes because I had a family history of it. My fasting blood sugar level was 118 and I was told I had borderline diabetes (an older term for prediabetes). I was told to lose weight and exercise but was not given any specific instruction on how to do it.

Several years later, I saw another doctor. My fasting sugar level was up to 200, and I was feeling weak and easily fatigued. I was referred to an endocrinologist. The diagnosis this time was mild diabetes. For the first time, I had a full lipid panel taken. The doctor said I had too little good cholesterol relative to my bad cholesterol, even though the total amount of cholesterol wasn't terribly high. The treatment for my cholesterol and diabetes was the same: diet and exercise.

At this point I was feeling confused, because although I had seen many doctors I still didn't know what I was dealing with or how to treat it, other than diet and exercise, which was not terribly successful. Frankly, I had been on one diet after another since I was fifteen years old and had never had much success at losing weight. And I didn't understand what was happening to me or how I should deal with it, so I couldn't do much to prevent it. The only thing I knew for sure was that I didn't want to end up like my mother.

I decided to find some answers and went to the bookstore. I read the Atkins diet book, I read Sugar Busters! *and I read a book entitled* Syndrome X. *I found my answers. I learned I had insulin resistance. I discovered if I kept my blood sugars in the normal range and took appropriate medications, along with (of course) the appropriate diet and exercise, I could lower my risk of ending up like my mother. I learned that exercise didn't mean running marathons. It just meant walking every day, with my son. I learned that pasta and rice and potatoes all increase my blood sugar levels just like sugar. And I found physicians who taught me how to take care of myself. I was started on a variety of medications to treat my blood sugar, insulin resistance, high blood pressure, and abnormal cholesterol levels. I have even lost 10 pounds and feel better all the time.*

There are still questions to be answered. My middle son was diagnosed with high cholesterol at age twelve. It improved with diet. My two oldest sons are in college now. They are thin and active. When should they be tested for insulin resistance? And how often? What should they be treated with, and when?

Most people who have diabetes have seen family members die from it. We live in fear that we will end up suffering as they did. We must face the heartbreak of wondering if we have passed this disease on to our children. With the right tools and information at the right time, you can compensate for family history and live well.

....

Lin's story exemplifies why you need to understand what insulin resistance is and what to do about it. Unfortunately Lin and her doctors didn't know enough to treat her warning signals early. Her mother was even less fortunate. You can do better.

How to Deal with Prediabetes

From a practical perspective you will want to take three proactive steps if you think that you might have insulin resistance and prediabetes. The first is to ask your physician to perform the tests I mentioned—fasting blood sugar, a lipid panel, blood pressure, and BMI based on height and weight.

If these results are not normal, the second step is to seek treatment (discussed in the next chapters). In many cases the treatments for most people who have insulin resistance will primarily target the risk for heart disease and will include a daily aspirin combined with specific medications to lower cholesterol and blood pressure. Sometimes, a diabetes-type medication is added for treating insulin resistance. But the overriding first choice for treatment is weight loss and exercise because almost everyone benefits from this. With diabetes, we're dealing with a genetic disorder brought on by a negative environment; adopting a healthier lifestyle makes a lot of sense.

The third and final step is to track your numbers over time. You want to be sure that your blood pressure and cholesterol numbers stay below the suggested target levels, but you will also want to follow your fasting blood sugar levels. If your fasting sugar starts at 102 and falls to 92 and stays below 100, that's great! But if it gradually increases, from 102 to 112 to 120, it means that your insulin resistance is getting worse and that you need to do something further to halt the progression to diabetes. As I've said before, the bad news is that this syndrome exists. But the really good news is that it is within your power to do something about it.

FIVE

CARBOHYDRATE-SENSITIVE (FORMERLY, REACTIVE) HYPOGLYCEMIA

Two hours after you have a doughnut and a glass of orange juice do you feel weak and shaky? Do you feel tired after eating a lunch of bread and pasta? If so, you may be feeling a change in your blood sugar levels due to eating too much refined carbohydrate.

People who have insulin resistance and prediabetes almost always seem to have these symptoms of hypoglycemia (low blood sugar) before they get diabetes. I think these symptoms should be on the list of warning signs for insulin resistance, prediabetes, and diabetes. However, because of the difficulty of defining and diagnosing this type of low blood sugar reaction it has been taken off the list of medical conditions associated with prediabetes and insulin resistance. Nevertheless, if you have hypoglycemic symptoms you should be tested for your diabetes risk, and treatment is generally the same in terms of diet, exercise, and certain medications that lower insulin resistance.

CARBOHYDRATE-SENSITIVE HYPOGLYCEMIA DEFINED

True hypoglycemia, a blood sugar level below 50 mg/dl, may or may not be found in patients with sensitivity to carbohydrates. Because of this, physicians have gotten away from calling the feeling of being shaky hypoglycemia, because it doesn't fit the medical definition for it. Yet it is a real phenomenon. In my experience many people who see me with a diagnosis of newly developed type 2 diabetes have had this sensitivity to carbohydrates for several years. In order to separate this feeling of hypoglycemia from the hypoglycemia that occurs when treating diabetes, I will call it "carbohydrate-sensitive" hypoglycemia, because it is a feeling of low or falling blood sugar after eating carbohydrates.

WHAT HAPPENS TO CARBOHYDRATES IN THE BODY?

When we eat carbohydrates, such as sugar, starch, pasta, and rice, our body makes insulin to bring blood sugar levels back to normal. This is a perfectly calibrated process, whereby the right amount of insulin is secreted to handle the increase of sugar in the blood. But when you are developing diabetes and have insulin resistance, sometimes your body makes too much insulin (it is trying to over-come the obstacle of the insulin resistance). This makes your body sense a rapidly falling blood sugar and it sends out alarm signals as though your blood sugar levels are becoming seriously low. This makes you react by wanting to eat more carbohydrate quickly, to treat the reaction and bring your blood sugar back up. Once this happens your sugar goes up and then swings back down again. While this is happening you can often feel drained and tired and this craving for more carbohydrates can make it hard to stick to a sensible diet. Your moods, fatigue, and hunger oscillate up and down; you never feel quite right, even though you're not really sick.

DIAGNOSING HYPOGLYCEMIA

Why Oral Glucose Tolerance Tests Are Not the Answer

There are many myths and misconceptions about diagnosing carbohydrate-sensitive hypoglycemia. First, it usually doesn't hap-pen during a glucose tolerance test—the test where you drink a sugary soda and the doctor measures blood sugar levels two to five hours afterward. Glucose tolerance tests are good for only two things. The first, and most common, is to diagnose disorders of *increased* blood sugar levels. These include diabetes, prediabetes, and gestational diabetes. The second, less common, use for a glu-cose tolerance test is to diagnose a condition of excess growth hormone, called acromegaly. Neither of these circumstances in-volves low blood sugar levels.

Testing for hypoglycemia was in vogue in the 1960s. At the time, very low levels of blood sugars were found in women who had glucose tolerance tests. After five hours the women would feel weak and shaky and would have blood sugars in the 40s. They were diagnosed with hypoglycemia. This may seem logical, but a smart researcher decided to test what was really happening. He did glucose tolerance tests on women without telling them their blood sugar levels. What he found was that there was no relationship between the blood sugar levels and symptoms. Some women had blood sugar levels in the 40s and no symptoms at all. In fact, it was discovered that young, active, healthy women may normally have blood sugar levels in the 40s and 50s and feel fine. The women who had symptoms of low blood sugar had symptoms at varying blood sugar levels—some at 70 mg/dl and others at 50. But the blood sugar levels and the symptoms were not necessarily related.

Some women had blood sugar levels in the 40s with no symptoms at all.

My experience leads me to conclude that there is, in fact, a reaction to sudden increases and falls in blood sugar levels. This may be due to too much insulin release, although it could be due to other hormones released by the stomach and other organs, as well. There are many hormones that are released from the intestines, some of which we have isolated and some of which are uncharacterized, that alter our physical and psychological responses to food. This science is in its infancy, but it is likely that someday these hormones will be recognized as being just as important as insulin in terms of regulating how food gets absorbed from our intestines, and how we feel after we eat certain types of food.

Making a Proper Diagnosis

To diagnose hypoglycemia, one must first rule out a serious cause such as an insulinoma (a tumor of the pancreas that causes the production of too much insulin) or other rare condition or disease, such as tumors of the peritoneum, adrenal insufficiency, kidney failure, or congestive heart failure. The best way to determine if hypoglycemia is present is to have you test your own blood sugar levels at home, first thing in the morning, so you know what your blood sugar level is when you wake up. You test your blood sugar levels at home with a small machine called a glucose meter. You can buy this from a drug store or get it from your physician's office. To test your sugar you need three things: a meter, strips to put into the meter to measure your blood sugar, and a lancing device to poke your finger for blood. To measure your sugar you prick your finger, which produces a drop of blood which you place on the glucose strip that is inserted into the meter. Usually it takes only five to twenty seconds to get the blood sugar reading. Your physician or educator can help you choose a meter and teach you how to use it correctly. Instructions for use also come inside the meter box, as does a lancet and a small number of strips. If the blood sugar level is below 60 mg/dl first thing in the morning it could be a sign of a more serious type of hypoglycemia.

To test your sugar you need three things: a meter, strips to put into the meter to measure your blood sugar, and a lancing device to poke your finger for blood.

You would also test your blood whenever you had symptoms of a low blood sugar reaction—which often happens after eating a high carbohydrate meal. Additionally, you'd test one or two times during the day when you don't have symptoms, say every day at four PM or at noon. This way, you learn what your blood sugars usually are. Keep a written data log, starting with writing down what your symptoms are and only then testing your blood sugar levels. Sometimes seeing a number that is low can make us think we are having symptoms of hypoglycemia when we are not. So writing down your symptoms before you test your blood sugar levels is the way to best tell if your symptoms are due to your blood sugar levels or not.

After a patient tests sugars for a week or two, I look at the written results. If the morning blood sugar level was below 60 or if it was less than 50 throughout the day, I will probably test for more serious causes of hypoglycemia, such as for the tumors mentioned earlier. If the patient's blood sugar levels were higher, or the symptoms less severe, I will probably prescribe treatment for carbohydrate-sensitive hypoglycemia. This would include following a diet described for prediabetes. In all cases, I would test for prediabetes and diabetes even though hypoglycemia is not always a symptom of prediabetes or diabetes. This would entail a fasting sugar level, fasting lipids, and a chemistry panel that includes kidney and liver function tests as well as thyroid function tests. These tests would be helpful not only in assessing whether or not there is prediabetes or insulin resistance, but also whether there are any kidney or liver abnormalities, both of which can cause low blood sugar reactions.

TREATMENT

If you are found to have carbohydrate-sensitive hypoglycemia, the key to treatment is to decrease how much simple carbohydrates you eat. This could include limiting refined sugar, fruit juice, flour, and/or rice. (This is all described in detail in chapter 7, on nutrition for prediabetes.) I also suggest patients eat frequent small snacks containing carbohydrate, protein, and fat. This helps regulate how quickly blood sugar levels rise in your system and also decreases the ensuing fall in blood sugar levels. There may not always be big increases or decreases in measured blood sugar levels. Often, seemingly small swings in blood sugar levels can make people feel tired, moody, irritable, or unable to fully concentrate.

There are people, too, who experience the blurred vision, headache, and shakiness of low blood sugar, usually before eating, because they have waited too long to eat. This may be a subjective sense of hypoglycemia that may or may not mean that something more serious exists. As noted, everyone with these symptoms should be tested for prediabetes, insulin resistance, and diabetes. The shakiness and blurred vision is not necessarily due to actual low blood sugar levels. More likely they relate to the fact that blood sugar levels are falling. *This is not science*—just my personal observation (and the observation of many others). I get these symptoms sometimes, too, so I avoid doughnuts and fruit juice. I also know I have a slight risk for diabetes, but there is not a blood test in the world that would prove anything; my labs are completely normal. I just control it by eating frequent small meals that are low in carbs as we describe in chapter 7.

Often, seemingly small swings in blood sugar levels can make people feel tired, moody, irritable, or unable to fully concentrate.

Nutrition and exercise are the first-line treatments for carbohydrate-sensitive hypoglycemia just as they are for treating the metabolic syndrome. Because weight loss and exercise improve insulin sensitivity and help to lower insulin levels, almost everyone I treat for carbohydrate-sensitive hypoglycemia feels better after they change their dietary patterns. In general, I recommend working with a nutritionist, but the suggestions in chapter 7 outline appropriate eating patterns for people with carbohydrate-sensitive hypoglycemia as well as for people with insulin resistance and prediabetes. In the same way, the use of drugs to decrease insulin resistance, such as metformin (Glucophage) and the glitazones, can help treat more severe symptoms of this type of hypoglycemia. Since this is not an approved use of these medications (these drugs are approved for treating diabetes only), you need to find a physician experienced in evaluating and treating people with hypoglycemia.

When I see a patient for evaluation of prediabetes, I also ask about symptoms of carbohydrate-sensitive hypoglycemia. These symptoms can be overlooked, in part because patients often get used to having it or they don't realize that it could be a sign of insulin resistance. One population where I see the problem with increasing frequency is overweight, at-risk adolescents who fall asleep at school after eating the typical high-carbohydrate kid breakfast of cereal, banana, milk, and toast. Adam's story below (which is actually a composite of various patients' stories) shows how much benefit there can be in identifying and treating this problem.

....

"He understood he could develop diabetes and wanted to do something about it."

Adam is a 240-pound sixteen-year-old high school student. He is bright and friendly and loves to draw political cartoons, which he publishes in his school newspaper. He makes people laugh. But Adam loves sweets and he hates to exercise. He is a video and computer game expert, but doesn't have any interest in playing soccer or running on the cross-country track team. His mother brought him to see me because there is a family history of diabetes and she was worried that he was at risk for getting diabetes, too. She also hoped that a fear of getting diabetes would motivate him to lose weight.

When I saw him he said he felt tired and unmotivated, particularly in school when he would feel weak and shaky in the middle of the morning. He would drink a soda or have a candy bar (or two) as a snack, which generally made him feel tired. Then he would eat lunch and would be exhausted by the time he returned home from school. I felt that many of these symptoms were due to carbohydrate-sensitive hypoglycemia.

I tested Adam's fasting blood sugar level and had a lipid panel done and found signs of metabolic syndrome. His fasting blood sugar level was elevated at 112 mg/dl (normal is less than 100 mg/dl) and his triglycerides were over 200 (normal is less than 150 mg/dl). He understood that this meant he could develop diabetes and heart disease and, much to his mother's relief, he wanted to do something about it.

His first treatment was to change his diet and increase his exercise. He met with a nutritionist who recommended that he switch from having a large bowl of cereal with milk and toast for breakfast to low-fat yogurt and string cheese. As soon as he did, he reported feeling more awake and alert at school. He changed his other meal choices as well, replacing refined or simple carbohydrates with healthier snacks, such as nuts, fresh fruit with peanut butter, or high-protein energy bars. Adam began to exercise, mostly walking, and gradually built up to forty-five minutes per day. Over six months he lost about thirty pounds. Not only did he tell me he felt better and better, he also markedly lowered his risk for getting early heart disease and diabetes.

....

....

SIX

FEMALE TROUBLES: INSULIN RESISTANCE, POLYCYSTIC OVARIAN SYNDROME, AND GESTATIONAL DIABETES

There are two issues unique to women that involve insulin resistance: polycystic ovarian syndrome (PCOS) and gestational diabetes (GDM). Both of these conditions were discussed briefly earlier, among risk factors for prediabetes or type 2 diabetes. If you are a woman and you haven't considered the questions outlined on pages 6–7, do so now. This chapter will arm you with exactly what you need to know if you have PCOS or are predisposed to gestational diabetes. Gentlemen readers may prefer to jump ahead to the next chapter, or read on to better understand (or impress) their wives or female friends.

POLYCYSTIC OVARIAN SYNDROME (PCOS)

A Simple PCOS Risk Test

1. Are you 40 pounds or more overweight (especially with central-body weight gain)?

2. Do you have a family history of type 2 diabetes?

3. Do you have irregular periods?

4. Is there above-average hair growth on your chin and upper lip?

5. Can you see a darkening of the skin around your neck or under your arms?

6. Have you been treated for infertility?

If you answered yes to question 3 and any other question, you could have PCOS and should read the information that follows.

Despite its mouthful of a name, polycystic ovarian syndrome (PCOS) is one of the conditions I most like to treat because I get to help my patients have babies. PCOS is probably the most common cause of infertility in the United States and can cause a decrease in menstrual periods, increased facial hair, acne, and other abnormalities. Polycystic ovarian syndrome means many ("poly") cysts on the ovaries, which really doesn't describe what causes it. The name was given to the condition long before we identified PCOS as a form of insulin resistance.

Women who are having trouble becoming pregnant often are referred to me. Their gynecologist wants an endocrinologist to test whether or not there are hormonal problems causing the infertility. I'm asked to check thyroid and hormone production, but in almost all of the cases the infertility I find is due to insulin resistance and PCOS, a disorder that can be caused by increased insulin levels.

PCOS often goes unrecognized. Not all PCOS is caused by insulin resistance. Because there is no one specific test for PCOS, we don't have exact numbers on its prevalence.[2]

But insulin resistance is the underlying problem in many cases. If you think you might have PCOS you should be sure to undergo complete testing for insulin resistance, as well as other causes for PCOS, which include obscure diseases such as adult-onset congenital adrenal hyperplasia, Cushing's syndrome, and tumors that secrete androgens.

PCOS causes irregular or absent menstrual cycles even more frequently than infertility, as well as acne, excessive facial hair, and a variety of other abnormalities. All can be corrected by treating the insulin resistance. If you have eight or fewer menstrual cycles per year, odds are that you have PCOS (unless you are on hormonal birth control or close to menopause). In some women, menstrual cycles stop completely. If treatment is working, normal cycles will return. A woman with PCOS probably is someone who started her periods a little bit later than other girls, and never settled into a completely normal pattern of cycles.

A common risk factor for having PCOS is being overweight. The other risks for having insulin resistance or prediabetes also come into play. Again, these are having a family history of diabetes or early heart disease, or belonging to high-risk ethnic groups. The troublesome conditions of high triglyceride, low HDL levels, and high blood pressure all are present in women who may develop PCOS.

Insulin Resistance and the Ovaries

The ovaries are a source of both male and female hormones. Women must have normally functioning ovaries in order to have normal hormone levels. If insulin resistance occurs, increased insulin levels, plus a number of other complex and difficult changes that we do not fully understand, can directly affect the ovaries.[3]

One of these effects is the formation of cysts on the ovaries. These cysts, filled with fluid, do not cause cancer, but they are clear evidence that insulin resistance is present. So, although finding ovarian cysts may show that you have PCOS, you can have PCOS without having ovarian cysts. Conversely, you can have cysts without having PCOS. As happens so many times in medicine, the condition was named before anyone realized what the syndrome truly was, or how many people might have it.

You can have PCOS without having ovarian cysts.
Conversely, you can have an ovarian cyst
without having PCOS.

When the balancing act of hormones is disrupted by insulin resistance and elevated levels of insulin, the "female" hormone estrogen and the "male" hormone testosterone are produced in the wrong proportions. Women with PCOS make too much free (not bound) testosterone. This higher level of testosterone leads to an increase in facial and chest hair. In severe cases, I have seen women who are losing the hair on their heads in a male pattern (from the front and sides) and who have increased muscle mass in their upper arms and chest. Extra testosterone also can cause acne and in very extreme cases a lower, "male"-sounding voice.

These abnormal hormone levels also inhibit normal ovulation (the release of the egg from the ovary into the fallopian tube that happens in the middle of the normal menstrual cycle). In addition to allowing pregnancy to occur, ovulation causes an increase in the hormone progesterone. Women with PCOS who do not ovulate have levels of progesterone that are too low. Progesterone is the hormone that balances estrogen and protects the uterus from endometrial cancer by causing monthly bleeding. When a patient is not trying to become pregnant, treating PCOS with birth control pills makes sense, because it keeps hormone levels in a safer, more normal range.

Skin Changes Caused by PCOS

Darkening of the skin around the neck and under the arms is a classic sign of PCOS. Patients will often tell me that they think they've become "dirty" and keep scrubbing at the skin around their neck to clean it off. But this is caused by a change in the pigment of the skin and won't come off even with a Brillo pad. This velvety darkening of the skin under the arms and around the nape of the neck is called *acanthosis nigricans*, which roughly translates as "dark skin." No one knows exactly what causes it, though it is associated with high insulin levels and colon cancer. Another PCOS-related condition is the development of skin tags. Skin tags are flaps of skin that generally are the same color as the rest of your skin, and occur in hot, moist body creases such as around the neck, under the arms or breasts, in the groin, or on the inside of the upper thigh. They tend to have narrow bases and can be as tiny as the head of a pin or can grow to one-half to one inch in size. They don't hurt unless they rub against your clothing and become irritated. We don't know what causes them, but probably high insulin levels play a role in their formation.

This velvety darkening of the skin under the arms and around the nape of the neck is called acanthosis nigricans, *which roughly translates as "dark skin."*

DIAGNOSING PCOS

As with many of the other types of insulin resistance, often it is the sum of all of our clinical findings that result in the diagnosis of PCOS. If a woman who is about 40 pounds overweight (especially in the central area of her body), has a family history of type 2 diabetes, and has irregular periods, an increase in hair growth on her chin and upper lip, and darkening of the skin around her neck walks into my office, I know she has PCOS. I always do blood work, though, as confirmation. This blood work starts with a fasting blood sugar level and fasting lipid panel, just as in all forms of diagnosing the metabolic syndrome. I also check kidney and liver function (liver function can be abnormal in some cases of insulin resistance). I will also do a pregnancy test, just to be sure. (It is more difficult to become pregnant with PCOS, but not impossible; sometimes the lack of periods is due to pregnancy.) Other hormones I measure include hormones related to the functioning of various endocrine organs, such as the adrenal, thyroid, and pituitary glands. I want to be sure they are okay and are not causing a disorder that is mimicking PCOS, which can happen.

In testing, I measure:

1. Prolactin level (made by the pituitary gland in the brain)

2. Thyroid function tests (hormones made by the thyroid gland)

3. Free and total testosterone (the male hormones that are present)

4. DHEA-S level (made by the adrenal glands)

If any one of these hormones is abnormal, further evaluation and treatment by an endocrinologist is required. Most times PCOS is simply PCOS, but it is important to confirm that everything hormonal is working the way it should. Most women with PCOS have experienced the gradual development of the syndrome over many years, usually since adolescence.

It is more difficult to become pregnant with PCOS, but not impossible.

Some physicians may wish to order an ultrasound of your ovaries. This is not necessary to make the diagnosis of PCOS, but it is sometimes helpful to know the extent of the problem. In my experience, heavily cystic ovaries are more likely to cause serious infertility.

Treatment of PCOS

Past and Present

There are multiple reasons to treat PCOS. The first is simple—most females don't want to look like males, and in particular would rather not have facial hair, go bald, or have acne. Women who want to have a baby and can't also need to treat their PCOS because the abnormal menstrual cycles brought on by PCOS mean difficulty conceiving (due to a lack of consistent ovulation). There are two other, perhaps less obvious, reasons to treat PCOS. With estrogen levels that are too high and progesterone levels that are too low, there is an increased risk for endometrial cancer in women with PCOS. Also, PCOS can be just like other forms of the metabolic syndrome and can lead to the development of heart disease and diabetes in susceptible individuals if it is not treated early.

In the past, doctors didn't really understand the relationship between insulin resistance and PCOS. Treatments were either cosmetic (to help with skin and hair growth) or surgical. Because many women with PCOS had ovaries filled with multiple cysts, it was felt that decreasing the number of cysts would help treat the PCOS. So surgeons did something called a wedge resection of the ovary—a procedure in which a wedge of ovarian tissue was cut out, leaving part of the ovary behind. The problem with this procedure? It rarely worked, because the cysts were caused by insulin re-sistance. If the insulin resistance isn't treated, the cysts come back. This procedure is done much less often than it once was, although an occasional person with excessive numbers of cysts may benefit.

Use of birth control pills works well to control some symptoms of PCOS, but in women with PCOS caused by insulin resistance this approach does not treat the underlying cause of the syndrome.

Another common treatment is to prescribe birth control pills to restart normal cycles. The birth control pills tend to shut off the ovaries and help give enough normal hormones so menstrual cy-cles begin. This lowers the increased risk for cancer. It also helps reduce the levels of male hormones. The best birth control pills are ones that contain 30 to 35 micrograms of ethinyl estradiol (the es-trogen component) and a progesterone, such as 0.5 milligrams of norethindrone, norgestimate, desogestrel, or drospirenone. All are progesterones that have few testosterone-like side effects. Among the popular birth control pills containing this combination (or a similar combination) are Yasmin, Alesse, and Levlen. Use of birth control pills works well to control some symptoms of PCOS, but in women with PCOS caused by insulin resistance this approach does not treat the underlying cause of the syndrome.

Diet and Exercise for the Insulin Resistance

The overall best way to treat PCOS is to lower insulin resistance. Just as with any other form of insulin resistance the treatment in-volves changing your diet, losing some weight (if you are over-weight), and increasing exercise. Some of my women patients have done amazingly well with this approach. As their lifestyle changes, they begin to have normal menstrual cycles, their skin gets better, and fertility comes back. In women not taking birth control pills, charting natural menstrual cycles is a great way to tell if the insulin resistance is decreasing. It is nature's way of telling us that insulin levels have fallen. Please be aware that normal menstrual cycles do not preclude PCOS. You can have normal (but anovulatory) menstrual cycles and yet have PCOS and be infertile. But in those without normal cycles, the return of cycles is a great way to measure progress.

You can have normal (but anovulatory) menstrual cycles and yet have PCOS and be infertile.

Medications for the Insulin Resistance

Some drugs designed for treating insulin resistance can also be used for treating PCOS. These drugs will be discussed in more detail in chapter 8, but lowering insulin resistance in PCOS can lower male hormone levels and help remedy the condition. The drug that has been studied most thoroughly is metformin. Metformin has been shown to help restore normal cycles and increase rates of ovulation, leading to improved fertility. Glitazone drugs, such as Actos (pioglitazone) and Avandia (rosiglitazone), lower insulin resistance very effectively. These drugs are newer than metformin, and are less well studied, but there are data to show these drugs work quite well at treating PCOS. I often prescribe metformin and a glitazone together, in order to optimally improve insulin resistance.

I treat patients with lifestyle change and medication, as much as is needed, until normal cycles return.

There are several issues related to using these drugs in treating PCOS. First, neither drug is approved for use in PCOS—they are treatments for type 2 diabetes, not for something that precedes diabetes. If we are using these drugs to treat PCOS, we must carefully follow patients and be clear on what the treatment goals are. In many cases I am trying to restore fertility, and that goal is fairly clear. I treat patients with lifestyle change and medication, as much as is needed, until normal cycles return. Once this happens, patients are free to conceive but must stop the metformin and/or glitazone im-

mediately upon conception. Some physicians have patients stop
these drugs a month or two before they try to conceive, which, if
possible, would be preferable. These drugs are not thought to be
dangerous during pregnancy, but that isn't known for sure.

---

*Women planning pregnancy should start taking 1 milligram
per day of folate, also known as folic acid, starting six
months prior to conception to help prevent defects in the
baby's nervous system (called neural tube defects).*

Prior to conception, women should speak with their gynecologist
or endocrinologist to inquire about any unusual risks to becoming
pregnant. Women planning pregnancy should start taking 1 milligram per day of folate, also known as folic acid, starting six
months prior to conception to help prevent defects in the baby's
nervous system (called neural tube defects).

If fertility does not come back with improvements in insulin
sensitivity, other approaches to the treatment of infertility may be
tried. Clomiphene citrate is often used to induce ovulation, and will
work in conjunction with treatments to reduce insulin resistance.
If clomiphene doesn't work, more complex approaches to restore
fertility can be tried under the supervision of a fertility specialist.

---

*I think it is very important that a woman decide from the
outset what her goals are and how to achieve them.*

Women who do not desire pregnancy need to know that once
they treat their insulin resistance they may become fertile (in some
cases, something they haven't been for a while). So if pregnancy isn't
desired, birth control should be used. Using glitazones with birth
control pills may lower the effectiveness of the birth control pills and
cause a risk for pregnancy. Another method of birth control may
need to be used. This should be discussed with your doctor. Treating
PCOS with metformin and/or a glitazone might cause real improvement in how a woman looks and feels thanks to an improvement in her hormonal balance. But this must be weighed against

the long-term use of drugs that could have unknown future risks. Metformin has been used worldwide since 1957, so we do have a lot of data on its use in people with diabetes.[4] This is why I think it is very important that a woman decide from the outset what her goals are and how to achieve them. These goals may include reduction of the physical changes (hair, skin) caused by PCOS, a stabilization or improvement of fasting blood sugar levels, a lowering of triglyceride levels, or an increase in HDL (good) cholesterol levels.

Cosmetic Options

In addition to the treatments for insulin resistance, there are other options for treating the sometimes slow-to-improve cosmetic issues that arise from PCOS.

1. For excessive facial hair, an oral drug called spironolactone can be used. This helps block the effect of testosterone on your hair follicles; dark male-pattern hairs don't grow. If you can't take this medication, or want to try something applied directly on the skin, there is Vaniqa (eflornithine hydrochloride cream 13.9%). This cream inhibits hair growth and must be applied to problem areas every day. Vaniqa also helps lessen the effects of male hormones on your hair follicles. Waxing, shaving, electrolysis, and laser hair removal works as it does in women without PCOS.

2. Balding can be more difficult to treat. First, have your thyroid checked (low thyroid function can cause hair loss). Topical Minoxidil can help some women the same way it helps balding men. Spironolactone is another option.

3. Acne and skin tags should be treated by a dermatologist, especially if the acne is not responding to over-the-counter treatments.

....

"If something does not seem right, it probably isn't."

Rebecca's is a great story with lessons for us all. She is trying to get pregnant as I write this book.

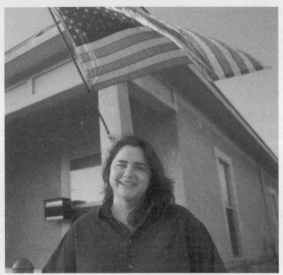

I first started my period at age thirteen. It took a few cycles before I began to realize I was irregular. I remember skipping the summer. It was months between cycles. This is not to say that I understood what irregular meant at that time. I just knew then that I wasn't having my period as often as the sex education class claimed I should. I didn't think much about it, especially since several of my friends seemed to be experiencing the same thing. We all just seemed to accept it and not ask questions.

I was born and raised in East Los Angeles. The majority of the population in my neighborhood is Latino (mostly Mexicans). I, being Mexican, know what it's like to be brought up in a culture where you just "accept" things that aren't what they should be. Which explains why my friends and I just accepted our irregular periods. To be honest, if a girl wasn't having a period on a normal basis, the first thing that most assumed was that she was pregnant. That was reason enough for most girls to keep quiet about her irregular periods. In addition, we wound up looking at irregular periods as a sort of gift. A woman's monthly visitor isn't particularly welcome, so skipping a month or two here and there wasn't so bad. Or so we thought.

As the years passed and we got older, many of us began to take oral contraceptives (the pill), which only masked the problems we were having with irregular cycles. In addition, I began to notice things on myself and even on a few close friends that seemed odd. But, again, I didn't question it. The things I noticed were dark patches of skin, excess facial and body hair growth, and thinning hair on the head. For years, I've recognized that something was wrong with me. I just didn't know what. There I was, twenty-something and growing skin tags, gaining weight, and having bouts of acne. Again, I was passive and didn't demand answers when I brought these issues to the attention of my doctors. Most were either not interested or all too quick to blame my weight for any problems that I was experiencing.

When my husband and I decided we wanted to consider starting a family, I stopped taking the pill. It was months before I had a period. I knew there had to be something wrong. I'd ask questions, but get prescriptions instead of answers. My general practitioner told me that I would probably have a period if I were to lose weight. Argh. I decided to start trying to get answers on my own. I learned about the importance of monthly cycles and decided it was probably best to go back to taking the pill for the sake of regulating my cycle.

A year later, I stopped the pill again and still no period. Somehow I was holding on to the notion that my body would eventually acclimate. I was wrong. I realized it was time to delve into books, magazines, and websites. Things were starting to add up and I knew I needed an answer. I went back to see my gynecologist and pushed for an ultrasound. My ob-gyn found cysts on my ovaries and finally diagnosed polycystic ovarian syndrome (PCOS). Hallelujah! For the first time ever, I knew why I should start taking the pill again.

It wasn't until I asked questions and demanded that ultrasound that I began to realize it doesn't matter where I live, or who I am, or what insurance I have. I should be asking questions and demanding answers. The answers are out there. You just have to push for them. I did. I also realized I needed an endocrinologist.

Thanks to the recommendation of a close friend, I wound up in the hands of an amazing endocrinologist. My first visit with her taught me so much about PCOS and what it has done and is doing to my body. I learned about the relationship between PCOS and insulin resistance. Blood tests later revealed I was, in fact, insulin resistant. I also learned about the connection between insulin resistance and diabetes and how important it was to focus on changing my lifestyle to prevent myself from getting type 2 diabetes. My mother has diabetes, which increases the likelihood that I could get diabetes.

I went back to researching and learned even more about PCOS. Everything began making sense. In addition to knowing what was wrong, I was also presented with options for treatment. My endocrinologist prescribed metformin to help control my blood sugar levels and I met with her nutritionist to work on a plan to help me incorporate necessary changes into a new lifestyle. I also began to make an effort to increase the amount of exercise that I get so that it, too, can become part of my life.

My diagnosis of PCOS and the resulting need to change my lifestyle may initially seem like bad news. However, once I educated myself about PCOS I realized that this should be looked at as a blessing rather than a curse. It was my look into the future. We rarely get an opportunity to change the future but the PCOS diagnosis gave me the chance. Armed with understanding and the support of my doctor, I fight on a daily basis. Some days are good, some aren't. All I know is that I will never give up or give in.

I began treatment nearly five months ago and have been fortunate enough to have lost 38 pounds thus far. Admittedly, it hasn't been easy. I know I'll fall down occasionally, but as long as I keep getting back up, that's all that counts.

You need to take control, ask questions, and be assertive. Don't let your heritage, background, or anything else keep you from wondering what's wrong with you. If something does not seem right, it probably isn't.

....

GESTATIONAL DIABETES

Gestational diabetes (GDM) is a temporary form of diabetes that may develop in the last part of pregnancy. Nearly every woman is tested at 24 to 28 weeks of pregnancy for the disorder, although some younger women (less than twenty-five years old) without any risk factors are not being screened. If you are reading this book, you probably have at least one risk factor for diabetes, and should be screened for gestational diabetes when you are pregnant, even if you're less than twenty-five years old.

Eight Risk Factors for Gestational Diabetes

1. Do you have a family history of type 2 diabetes (in a mother, father, sister, brother, or grandparent)?

2. Are you overweight (BMI greater than 25)?

3. Have you had a baby weighing 9 pounds or more?

4. Are you a member of a high-risk ethnic group, particularly American Indian, African American, Latino, South or East Asian, Pacific Islander?

5. At birth, were you either large (greater than 9 pounds) or small (less than 6 pounds)?

6. Do you have PCOS?

7. Have you had an unexplained fetal loss during pregnancy, or a child born with a malformation?

8. Are you older than twenty-nine?

Lists are not screening tests. If you have any of these risk factors you are a candidate for gestational diabetes and should be sure to read the rest of this chapter.

Insulin Resistance During Pregnancy

The rise in blood sugar levels associated with gestational diabetes is due to increased insulin resistance. Most women are tested for GDM during pregnancy, so it usually is picked up and treated. After pregnancy, however, women who have had GDM are at high risk for developing diabetes in the future. As with all other forms of insulin resistance, early detection can lead to treatment and prevention of diabetes. This is why it is so crucial to understand what insulin resistance is and how to keep it from developing into diabetes in the future.

When a woman is pregnant, her entire body is programmed to feed the baby growing inside her. Sugar is a basic fuel for the baby and freely passes through the placenta. A developing baby needs sugar to grow. Hence, the placenta makes its own hormones that increase insulin resistance during pregnancy. In an odd way, the increased insulin resistance seems to increase the sugar that is directed to the baby and decrease the amount taken up by the muscles and liver. This insulin resistance rises sharply in the last part of pregnancy.

If risk factors for diabetes are present or an early case of the metabolic syndrome exists, you may already be experiencing some insulin resistance going into pregnancy. Therefore, when the placenta makes pregnancy hormones, the body can't handle the added stress. This causes blood sugars to rise, and a pregnant woman to develop this temporary form of diabetes called gestational diabetes. Amazingly, in a routine pregnancy, insulin levels may need to increase threefold to keep the mother's blood sugar levels in the normal range. That's a lot of stress on the pancreas. No wonder some women need treatment for diabetes during pregnancy.

Understanding the Risk of Gestational Diabetes

The primary thing to know about GDM is that both you and your baby are likely to be fine as long as you stay in close touch with your health care team and keep your sugar levels in the normal range. Diabetes that is present when pregnancy starts (in women who have type 1 or type 2 diabetes *before* they get pregnant) can affect the development of the baby. This is discussed in chapter 17. By the time GDM usually is seen, the baby is already formed; it has arms and legs, a heart and brain. The extra sugar makes the baby grow too big and causes its newly formed pancreas to work overtime. If the mother's blood sugar levels are not brought down to normal, babies greater than 9 pounds are born (this is called macrosomia). These bigger babies are much harder to deliver and may develop low blood sugar reactions, jaundice, and a low blood calcium level during the first week of life. Normally these problems don't persist, and the baby is fine.

Big babies and small babies are at the highest risk for getting diabetes.

Please note that there also is a correlation between GDM and the development of diabetes in the child later in life because the mothers are at risk for diabetes as well, and diabetes is inherited. Big babies and small babies are at the highest risk for getting diabetes. The large babies caused by GDM also mean a higher chance of birth trauma and other serious problems, including death.

In my East Los Angeles Diabetes Center, there is a pattern of Latino women with gestational diabetes and poor prenatal care who deliver babies weighing 10, 11, even 12 pounds. Though most of these babies are healthy, there is no reason to chance a difficult delivery.

Testing for Gestational Diabetes

The first test for gestational diabetes is a glucose tolerance test. You drink about half a container of special sweet cola or orange drink. Then, your blood sugar is tested an hour later. This is called a screening test, which means it is used to pick up the possibility of GDM. If the blood sugar level is greater than or equal to 140 during the screening test, a more complete diagnostic test is required. For this second test, you drink the entire bottle of cola or orange drink. Blood sugar level is measured before the test, and then one, two, and three hours later.

When two or more of the tested blood sugar levels are higher than the guideline numbers below, gestational diabetes is present:

Fasting	Greater than 95 mg/dl
One hour after	Greater than 180 mg/dl
Two hours after	Greater than 155 mg/dl
Three hours after	Greater than 144 mg/dl

These are the strictest guidelines for gestational diabetes. As with many things in medicine, there is some debate as to which levels are the most accurate for diagnosing gestational diabetes. Since you don't want to take any chances when it comes to your health or the health of your baby, I'd recommend using these levels.

Treatment of Gestational Diabetes

If you are diagnosed with GDM, you need to immediately get treatment with close follow-up. Most communities have good prenatal health programs that you can join. In California, our program is called Sweet Success. As a society we seem to do a much better job of providing resources for gestational diabetes than we do for the treatment and prevention of type 2 diabetes, probably because everyone loves a baby. If your blood sugar levels are very high during pregnancy, your doctor may immediately start you on insulin. Women with GDM and lower blood sugar levels begin with a trial treatment of diet and exercise. In either case, you should meet with a nutritionist to learn how to eat appropriately for GDM and then with a diabetes educator (who could be the nutritionist) to teach you how to test your blood sugar levels. You should also work closely with your obstetrician to discuss approaches to exercise. You don't want to start rigorous physical activity halfway through pregnancy, although some increase in exercise is often good for you when your pregnancy is going well.

Most women treat their gestational diabetes through diet and exercise, but 15 percent will need insulin.

Reporting blood sugar numbers to a health care provider at least once a week will be required. Unfortunately, in pregnancy we usually ask you to test your blood sugar levels more often—before each meal and again one to two hours after, plus at bedtime. You fortunately only have to do this for about twelve weeks, which means that there's an end in sight.

Because insulin resistance will continue to increase in your body, it is possible that over time blood sugar levels will rise (in spite of diet and exercise) and you will need insulin. Most women treat their gestational diabetes through diet and exercise, but 15 percent will need insulin. The insulin is started when your fasting blood sugar level rises to above 90 mg/dl and/or your blood sugar rises to greater than 120 mg/dl one hour after eating. These are much more stringent values than we apply to nonpregnant patients, but tight blood sugar control in pregnancy is clearly beneficial to both mother and baby.

Your doctor will follow you more closely during the pregnancy, particularly in the final weeks. If it is thought the baby is having trouble or your gestational diabetes is not well controlled, your obstetrician may need to deliver the baby early. (This depends upon the baby's lungs being adequately mature.) Once your baby is born, it will be checked for low blood sugar levels. Low blood sugar can be caused by overactivity of the baby's beta cells in the womb, when they were required to keep up with the extra sugar received from the placenta. If the blood sugars are too low, the baby may need to stay in a neonatal intensive care unit for a day or two, until his or her sugar levels are normal. The baby also will be checked for excessive jaundice or other metabolic problems potentially caused by gestational diabetes.

As soon as the baby is delivered, gestational diabetes goes away.

After Your Baby Is Born

As soon as the baby is delivered, gestational diabetes goes away. If you were taking insulin during the pregnancy, chances are you won't need it anymore. A woman occasionally has "regular" (type 2) diabetes diagnosed during pregnancy that persists. Fortunately, this is rare. What doesn't go away in women who have had gestational diabetes is the risk for developing diabetes in the future. Up to half of the women who have had gestational diabetes will develop diabetes as they get older. If you had gestational diabetes with one pregnancy, you are quite likely to develop it with future pregnancies. Therefore, don't put diabetes completely out of your mind once you have delivered your baby.

It is recommended that six weeks after you deliver your baby you return to your doctor for another glucose tolerance test (one in which blood samples are drawn at baseline and two hours later). This will allow your doctor to determine whether or not you still have diabetes or impaired glucose tolerance. However, this test is only a one-time test and your risk for developing type 2 diabetes will continue to increase each year. You must monitor yourself throughout your life, as do people with the metabolic syndrome, because you can prevent the development of diabetes in the same way that anyone else can—through lifestyle change and, in some cases, medication. Also remember that children of mothers who had gestational diabetes are at increased risk for developing diabetes themselves. Therefore, encouraging a healthy diet and exercise may be extra beneficial for these children.

Insulin Resistance in Women

PCOS and GDM are two forms of insulin resistance that are seen in women. Although both of these conditions must be recognized and treated during childbearing years, it also is important to remember that they increase the risk for type 2 diabetes later on. Women are lucky in a way. Their female hormones are altered by insulin resistance in a manner that provides warning signals about future risk. Men don't have such a sign for possible diabetes. But many women aren't aware of what PCOS is or that it is a treatable form of insulin resistance. All people with insulin resistance require ongoing follow-up to be certain there is no further decline in their insulin levels; such monitoring allows you to catch problems early, when they can be effectively treated. I see many women with newly diagnosed type 2 diabetes who had gestational diabetes or delivered a big baby and had no idea they were at risk for developing diabetes. The key is to understand your risk and then to work to modify your lifestyle to prevent future diabetes onset.

Women are lucky in a way. Their female hormones are altered by insulin resistance in a manner that provides warning signals about future risk.

For any condition associated with insulin resistance, whether it is PCOS, gestational diabetes, prediabetes, or type 2 diabetes, the approach to nutrition and exercise is similar. The one exception is gestational diabetes; pregnancy may require exercise to be more limited and a nutritional assessment needs to be done to provide appropriate nutrition for mother and baby. However, eating a lower carbohydrate diet, with less refined food and more fresh fruits and vegetables, is healthy for everyone. In the next chapter, my nutritionist and I discuss how we teach patients to change their habits to establish a lifetime pattern of good nutrition and health.

SEVEN

CREATING HEALTHY HABITS: A SIMPLE APPROACH TO NUTRITION AND EXERCISE FOR PREVENTING DIABETES

First of all, *do not skip this chapter.* I understand that many of you have struggled with your weight for years and have yet to make exercise part of your normal routine. But it's never too late to start. There are no new gimmicks or tricks that can magically help you lose weight and keep it off. Long-term success comes from learning to adopt new, healthier patterns in your life. I teach my patients the science of eating and exercising in a way that suits their own personal preferences. We work together on establishing lifestyles they can live with. And our goals can be small, especially at first. Did you know that losing only a small amount of weight, say 15 pounds, can work wonders in preventing diabetes?

It is hard to learn everything about nutrition all at once. When we first meet with you at our clinic, we have you describe a typical day, telling us what you like to eat and don't like to eat. We then list five or six choices for each meal (that is, specific healthy suggestions for breakfast, lunch, and dinner with two small snacks in between). We also try to help you find time in your day for exercise, scheduling when and planning how you will exercise, rather than just telling you to join a gym and go from there.

After the first session, we try to help you become an expert in nutrition, or at least expert enough to make good choices. To understand nutrition you will need to learn about the different types of fat, carbohydrate, and protein, and how to combine these foods in a healthy way in your diet. Another critical concept is that of portion size—in our super-sized society it is important to learn what a healthy portion actually looks like.

This chapter begins to explore some of the issues surrounding nutrition and exercise, particularly as they relate to prediabetes. Chapter 10, which focuses on type 2 diabetes, goes into more detail about the elements of nutrition. The information in chapter 10 complements the suggestions made here, particularly because the diet recommendations for people with prediabetes and type 2 diabetes are essentially identical. While some repetition from section to section is unavoidable, please keep in mind that the nutrition plans for the various diabetes types do differ somewhat. Finally, in chapter 17, carbohydrate counting is described, which is essential if you take insulin or want a more advanced knowledge of nutrition.

PROOF THAT WEIGHT LOSS REALLY MATTERS

We are fortunate to have recent results of studies done in China, Finland, and the United States that prove that diet and exercise can prevent the development of type 2 diabetes. In these studies, the most telling of which is detailed below, all the patients had impaired glucose tolerance, a form of prediabetes. These patients were already at higher-than-normal risk for developing diabetes. In each and every one of the studies, diet and exercise reduced the risk for developing diabetes by about half. That could translate to five to ten years of extra, healthy life.

Reviewing the Diabetes Prevention Program

The Diabetes Prevention Program (DPP) study was conducted in the United States from 1997 to 2001. This was a big, national study, funded in part by the National Institutes of Health. Investigators in this study were located all around the country, so every region, ethnic group, and body size and shape was represented among the 3,234 people randomly chosen to participate. These people were placed into one of four groups. For the purpose of illustrating the benefits of diet and exercise, we'll focus on the one thousand patients whose lifestyle was modified. These subjects were compared to another group of one thousand that received no treatment whatsoever (the control or "placebo" group). (In the next chapter I will focus on the two groups that were treated with diabetes-prevention medication.)

Participants in the group that received the lifestyle treatment were taught how to eat a healthy diet. They attended sixteen education sessions over the first twenty-four weeks and afterward were contacted monthly. They were taught about diet, exercise, self-monitoring, goal setting, and problem solving. The first step toward weight loss was to have the subjects adjust their diets to lower the amount of fat they ate to 25 percent of their calorie intake. If that didn't work, participants were given a calorie goal to help them reduce further. The weight loss targets were modest—approximately 7 percent of an individual's body weight (which in most cases was a target of 7 to 21 pounds). Of equal importance to the weight loss was the expectation of maintaining it.

The first step toward weight loss was to have the subjects adjust their diets to lower the amount of fat they ate to 25 percent of their calorie intake.

To help patients reach their goals they had access to an individual lifestyle coach, who helped encourage them to lose weight and keep it off. Patients were weighed at routine follow-up visits, and were encouraged to track their weight at home. They were invited to attend periodic motivational campaigns and group walking events, as well as annual refresher classes. If you want to find out the specific details of the DPP Lifestyle program, all of the manuals are available on the Internet at http://www.bsc.gwu.edu/dpp/manuals.htmlvdoc.

Patients in the DPP were also encouraged to exercise thirty minutes per day at least five days per week. In addition to meeting with educators for exercise instruction, participants were provided the tools they needed (such as athletic shoes and exercise equipment) to help them reach the study targets. At this point you are probably thinking that with this much help, losing weight and exercising would be easy. In fact, it wasn't and never is, which is why constant support and encouragement are needed to help along the way.

The DPP study lasted for three years. As with many diet and exercise changes, there was early success. The first year patients lost, on average, 15 pounds (see the graph below). Over the next two years their weight crept up a few pounds, but patients in the lifestyle treatment group were still thinner than those in the control group. Approximately 750 of the 1,000 participants were able to exercise more than they had before and many approached the goal of exercising thirty minutes per day, five days per week, with the most common form of exercise being simple brisk walking.

What happened in the DPP study was so phenomenal that the study was stopped one year early—the NIH study monitoring board felt that the results were so positive, compelling, and conclusive that no further research was needed. What were these compelling results? It was demonstrated that the loss of about 15 pounds reduced the

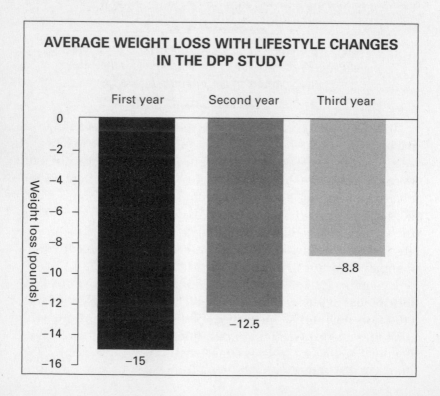

AVERAGE WEIGHT LOSS WITH LIFESTYLE CHANGES IN THE DPP STUDY

risk for developing diabetes by more than half (58 percent)! This is an astonishing, clear, and significant result. And when you consider that the alternative is diabetes, 15 pounds really isn't all that much to lose.

The loss of about 15 pounds reduced the risk for developing diabetes by more than half.

What the DPP Results Mean to You

The challenge of the DPP is twofold: lose some weight, and keep it off. If you do nothing now, chances are you will join the average American who gains 2 pounds per year. (Which requires that you eat a mere 25 extra calories per day in excess of what you burn.) This cumulative increase in your weight would lead to an increased burden on your pancreas and, should you have the genes for diabetes, a guaranteed future diagnosis of type 2 diabetes.

Although exercise is good for you, and has many health benefits, weight loss was the real key to preventing diabetes in the DPP study. Your body reacts to the extra weight by increasing the insulin resistance in your body. This means your body needs to release more and more insulin from the beta cells in the pancreas to keep the blood sugar levels normal. In some people the beta cells can keep working overtime for a lifetime. In others (for example, those with a family risk for diabetes), the beta cells stop being able to keep up with the demands placed on them and insulin levels fall. When the insulin level falls, blood sugar levels rise and diabetes sets in. Weight reduction lowers the stress on the beta cells. Your body needs to make less insulin because there is less resistance. The beta cells are then able to make enough insulin to keep blood sugar levels in check.

Researchers will spend years pouring over all of the data that was created in the Diabetes Prevention Program study. But for our purposes, it is enough to know that the benefits of weight loss extended throughout every ethnic group, and that older patients (greater than sixty years of age) got diabetes at an even lower rate than their younger counterparts. No matter what your age or race, this represents a positive road map to a healthier life.

THE NUTS AND BOLTS OF WEIGHT LOSS FOR DIABETES PREVENTION

Making changes in your diet can be very challenging because eating is not something we can completely avoid—or want to. Food is everywhere we look. We see it in television commercials, in magazines, and on billboards. We can buy it everywhere, especially processed or junk foods: in grocery stores, fast food restaurants, gas stations, movie theaters, and in vending machines down the hall. Even hospital cafeterias aren't always model sources of good nutrition.

The best aspect of the type of "diet" that my clinic recommends is that there is no restrictive diabetic diet, no special foods you have to eat. As someone with prediabetes, you can still enjoy your favorite foods on this diet. You just can't have them every day and you probably will have to eat slightly less of them than before. Did you know that if you ate just three bites less of your favorite fast food hamburger, you would be eliminating 100 calories a day from your diet? And eliminating even 100 calories a day is a start in preventing weight gain.

Eliminating even 100 calories a day is a start in preventing weight gain.

So if you can learn not to "clean your plate" as your mother taught you, but rather to leave a little bit behind at every meal, you would go a long way toward decreasing the excess calories you may eat every day.

Pairing healthy eating with walking for fifteen minutes more per day can also help you turn the corner toward health. I recommend the website http://www.americaonthemove.org/. This site has great strategies for increasing exercise and decreasing the number of calories eaten per day—ideas to help anyone become (and stay) thinner and more fit. One tip is to buy a step counter and establish a pattern of walking two thousand more steps a day with an ultimate goal of ten thousand steps per day. There are many ways to increase your walking. Park a little farther away from the mall, or take the stairs instead of the elevator. My personal strategy is having a treadmill in front of my TV so I can watch my favorite TV shows while I exercise.

Later in the chapter we'll have more to say about exercise, but for now here are other simple ways to benefit more from your normal activities.

Easy Ways to Increase Your Daily Steps and Exercise

- Park in the farthest corner of any parking lot, or a block or two away from work.

- Walk up and down the stairs instead of using the elevator.

- Walk beside, not on, moving sidewalks and escalators.

- Put a piece of exercise equipment in front of the television and try to watch only when you are exercising.

- Every thirty minutes take a "movement break." Walk around your building or house, walk up and down a flight of stairs or two, do jumping jacks, or just stretch your muscles.

- When ferrying luggage or grocery bags between your car and house, for example, carry fewer items each trip. Walk briskly back and forth as many times as you can until the task is completed.

- Use weekends or days off to go to places where you can get exercise. Walk around the zoo, through a park, or in a shopping mall. Go on a walking tour of your city. Bicycle or walk through your neighborhood. Walk to your local store or to visit a friend.

Revise your attitude toward exercise so you find ways to walk and expend energy at every opportunity. A very rich man I know always finds ways to save money. He loves to save a dollar by going to a discount store, even though he has millions to spend. I think it is his attitude of endless thriftiness that led him to his fortune. Applying this same savvy approach to exercise also can pay big dividends. Each time you wait for an elevator to go up only one or two floors or are drawn to eat a rich dessert, think again. Use your body. Expend extra energy. Eat a little less. A few more steps here and there, 100 calories not eaten, will add up to better health. However, be careful not to fall into the trap of saying, "I exercised, therefore I can eat more." If you want to *lose* weight you must eat fewer calories than you burn. Once you are in the weight *maintenance* phase, exercising allows you to eat more calories than if you weren't working out.

The Weight Loss and Regain Roller Coaster

Chances are you've struggled with your weight ever since you stopped racing around as a teenager. You've tried lots of diets. They all work for a while, but inevitably you go back to your old habits, because it's easier and feels more familiar. And, darn, weight loss is so slow it becomes incredibly frustrating. Right?

Deep down, we all really want an easy answer. But by now you likely know that it is time, at last, to change your habits for good and for a lifetime. When you adopt new patterns you will change for good. But as long as you feel you're on a diet you will struggle. You must stop feeling endlessly deprived. When you completely adopt a new relationship with food, you will win the weight battle.

In the context of prediabetes and insulin resistance there is a 15- to 20-pound "weight gap"—the amount most people need to lose to remain healthy.

At this point, I want to be absolutely clear that no one is passing judgment on you. I do not think that fat is bad, ugly, a sign of moral sloth, or anything else negative. I know a lot of attractive, functional, happy overweight people. But in the context of prediabetes and insulin resistance there is a 15- to 20- pound "weight gap"—the amount most people need to lose to remain healthy. And it is the effort to lose that weight, as a form of medical therapy, that I want to focus on.

I see hundreds of patients embark on the path of trying to lose weight and increase their physical activity. Almost all of them succeed initially. But our role models should be the people who lose weight and really do manage to stay thinner. The one thing common to those who succeed long term is that they have found a way to incorporate new patterns into their lives in comfortable ways and realize that their old habits don't work for them. Most don't end up "skinny." They will never be fashion models in *Vogue* (who of us ever will?), but they are healthier people because of the changes they've made.

I wish I could figure out what psychological button gets triggered that allows those with weight loss success stories to adapt to new eating approaches and not feel deprived. Almost all have tried to lose weight many times over the years, and have either not been successful or have lost weight and gained it back. And although I think the psychological reasons for overeating are complex (and I encourage patients to see a therapist when they need help dealing with their psychological issues), it seems that patients who succeed long term follow a form of behavioral modification. In other words, they establish new patterns of eating and stick to them with little deviation. A motivation to change is essential. I think that comes from an inner desire to be healthier. Our weight loss role models have incorporated a new intellectual and emotional reality for themselves that feels right and helps them eat less.

A motivation to change is essential. I think that comes from an inner desire to be healthier.

Is One Diet Better Than Another?

Studies show that many diets work. I do not advocate any one particular diet program, book, or plan, although a number of good ones are available. Whatever approach resonates with you personally is the one you should try. Many of my patients like the South Beach diet, which seems healthy from a nutritional perspective. Another excellent book is *Five-Factor Fitness* by Harley Pasternak, which gives specific examples of both healthy eating *and* exercise routines. As I will discuss below, I think that patients with diabetes and prediabetes do best if they reduce the amount of carbohydrate they eat and learn how to introduce more healthy, unrefined foods into their diet. Many researchers are looking at the pros and cons of various diets. What we know already is that the high-protein, low-carbohydrate Atkins-type diets and the less-carbohydrate-restricted Weight Watchers approach produce weight losses similar to those seen in the DPP. But with Atkins (particularly the strict Atkins plan), once people start eating carbohydrates again or deviate too far from the structured diet, they put the weight back on. Since sustained weight loss is our goal, this makes Atkins-type diets less appealing. The weight regain may be less true for Weight Watchers because of the ongoing follow-up and support to maintain weight loss, and because its plan allows a broader variety of food types. Other support groups, like Overeaters Anonymous, can be very effective for certain patients.

Sustained weight loss is our goal.

In addition to weight control programs, there are also many excellent books on weight loss. Since new books come out so frequently, it is hard to comment on which one is best at any given time. Be cautious of the "science" used to back up specific diet plans since it tends to be slanted to justify whatever the book's approach to weight loss might be. But overall, these diets do help you lose weight at least in the short term because they limit your food choices, thereby limiting your caloric intake.

There are successful medically supervised liquid protein fasting types of diets, but as with any diet where nutrition choices are extremely limited to produce weight loss, many people gain back the weight they lose (and more) after they return to eating regular food. A variation of this approach is to drink a meal replacement (such as Choice, Glucerna, or Slim-Fast) for breakfast and lunch, and then eat a healthy dinner. Here is an example of how this works into your day:

A Sample Day (1,200 Calories)

8:00   Meal replacement product

10:00   Fruit

12:30	Meal replacement, steamed vegetables or salad
4:00	1 ounce peanuts
6:00	Healthy dinner: 3 ounces protein, ¾ cups brown rice, 2 cups vegetables
8:00	Fruit

This is a way to limit food choices for part of the day, while learning new patterns for eating dinner that you eventually work into the rest of your daily meals.

Some people opt for a surgical approach to reducing obesity. This can be very effective, but has its own share of risks and benefits. If you choose this approach, be sure to see a surgeon who does the procedure frequently. I suggest researching the different types of surgical weight-reduction procedures to find the one best suited to you. And note that many insurance companies require documentation of past participation in standard weight reduction programs without sustained success. Consult your nutritionist to help you document your history.

A Healthy Approach to Weight Loss

The best thing you can do is to find a nutritionist you can work with, either individually or as part of a group. A good nutritionist can help fashion a meal plan that works for you, customized to your own particular tastes and style of eating. He or she will help guide you toward whatever methods of weight loss seem most promising. You want to choose a nutritionist who is not judgmental about your weight. You should never be made to feel uncomfortable about "failure." You know better than anyone what you've been eating. If weight loss were easy, we'd all be lean and lithe. Assemble a team that not only provides support, encouragement, and education, but exhibits a willingness to work with you regardless of whether or not you are able to make lasting changes in your diet.

If weight loss were easy, we'd all be lean and lithe.

The Best Time to Change Is Now

I have learned that not all patients have the same readiness to commit to changes in lifestyle. Almost every new patient initially tells me that he or she is ready to change everything for the sake of their health, but over time that enthusiasm can quickly fade. Knowledge of nutrition has very little to do with whether or not you will be able to change your behaviors or habits. What is important is *attitude*, the openness to change. The list below outlines the five basic levels of readiness to change nutritionists and diabetes educators have learned to recognize in their clients.[5]

The Five Stages of Change

1. *No way:* Having no intention of taking action in the foreseeable future.

2. *Preparation:* Intending to take action in the foreseeable future.

3. *Good intentions:* Intending to take action in the next thirty days.

4. *Action:* Actively practicing the behavior and actions necessary to reach your personal goal level for less than six months.

5. *Maintenance:* Continuing new, healthy habits for six months or more.

A proven condition for success is at least being in the "preparation" stage, when you have considered the groundwork necessary to begin making behavioral changes. If you are not in the right stage, your success is bound to be limited. Most patients who start diets stop within two to four weeks, largely because they don't get the right advice at the right time to create lasting change. So it is important to work with someone who can help you reach the preparation level in order to succeed at lifestyle change. The most powerful motivator is the inner voice that comes from within you, from a place of true commitment, that reminds you to be healthier and improve your life. You can't make major lifestyle changes because your husband wants you to lose weight or your kids are bugging you. Probably doing it just so you can fit into a bikini for the summer isn't enough, either. The desire has to start and end with being good to yourself, taking care of yourself in a way that will have lasting benefits. That way, you can override any psychological or physiological connections you have with food that keep you eating too much.

The most powerful motivator is the inner voice that comes from within you, from a place of true commitment, that reminds you to be healthier and improve your life.

CREATING A HEALTHY LIFESTYLE

Once you have come to the point where you think you are ready to make a lasting change, follow the steps below to begin establishing a healthier lifestyle. But remember that patients with insulin resistance have a harder time losing weight than those who don't. The genes that go along with the metabolic syndrome are the genes that help you survive famine, which means that when you start eating less your body tries extra hard to hang on to your fat. When a person with type 2 diabetes goes on a diet it is much harder for him or her to lose weight compared to someone without diabetes. Don't get discouraged and don't compare your progress to anyone else's. As long as you eat fewer calories and exercise more, you will lose weight. And although I have lots of people say to me that they "don't eat much" or that they're getting older and gaining weight even though they've always eaten the same way, it doesn't matter because if someone is overweight then the number of calories they are eating is too much. It probably isn't fair that some people seem to be able to eat so many calories compared to others. Despite your metabolism you can lose weight as long as you eat fewer calories than you burn. It really *is* that simple.

Don't get discouraged and don't compare your progress to anyone else's.

———

*Despite your metabolism you can lose weight as long as
you eat fewer calories than you burn.*

———

To lose a pound, you need to burn 3,500 calories. The reverse is
true of gaining a pound: consume those 3,500 calories again—and
don't burn them off—and you are up 1 pound. This applies no
matter who you are. I strongly believe we in America have gotten
used to thinking we need to eat more food than we really do. So
become an expert in estimating serving sizes. That way, you can
figure out how much to eat at any meal. A good website for estimating the food and calorie composition of your diet is www.fitday.com.
   The list below condenses the information in the pages that follow, which contain commentary on each of the twelve keys.

Twelve Keys to a Healthy Lifestyle

1. Understand carbohydrates, fats, and proteins and how to
   balance your meals.

2. Engage in daily physical activity.

3. Learn about proper portion sizes.

4. Use the plate method to balance meals and control portions.

5. Keep food consumption records.

6. Clean up your food environment.

7. Learn to know your hunger.

8. Eat and drink small amounts often, so you never feel too
   hungry.

9. Don't be a slave to the scale.

10. Plan your meals for a week at a time.

11. Eat more fruits and vegetables.

12. If you smoke, quit!

1. Understand Carbohydrates, Fats, and Proteins and How to Balance Your Meals

Up until now, we have talked about motivation and change, what it takes mentally and emotionally to lose weight. Now it's time to talk physical specifics, beginning with the classification of the foods we eat. There are three major food categories: carbohydrates, fats, and proteins. We need all three to live.

No matter what carbohydrate goes into your mouth, all are broken down in your intestines and enter your bloodstream as glucose, a form of simple sugar.

Carbohydrate is the primary source of sugar in your blood. It is the only fuel your brain can use and it powers your muscles and other organs. Carbohydrate comes in many forms. The simplest and most obvious form is table sugar and candy. More complex forms are the starches that most people don't consider to be sugar, such as breads and cereals, pasta, rice, and potatoes. Fruits, vegetables, milk, and yogurt are mostly carbohydrates as well, although dairy products also contain protein and fat.

No matter what carbohydrate goes into your mouth, all are broken down in your intestines and enter your bloodstream as glucose, a form of simple sugar. The more fiber a food has, like high-fiber uncooked fruits and vegetables, the slower the sugar is absorbed. The simple sugars are immediately absorbed. Your body stores sugar mainly in your muscles and liver. It also is collected in fat (but in a different form). Because sugar is vital to the functioning of your body, sugar is made from protein if you don't eat any carbohydrate. When a person without diabetes is on a high-protein diet, the body's blood sugar levels don't fall; it simply converts protein to sugar. If enough protein isn't eaten to keep glucose levels high, your body will break down muscle to make the glucose it requires. In other words, muscle is a stored form of protein. Fat, however, can never be reconverted to sugar.

Protein is a building block for muscles, skin, and hair—basically all our body parts. Protein comes from animal sources (beef, lamb, poultry, fish, pork), vegetable sources (soybeans, lentils, split peas, grains), nuts (the best are walnuts, almonds, and peanuts), dairy (milk, cheese, yogurt), and eggs. Depending on the source of the protein, it is accompanied by more or less saturated fat and cholesterol. High amounts of fat make meat taste better (like a well-marbled steak), but this is probably the worst form of protein for you to eat. Poultry, fish, legumes and grains, nuts, low-fat dairy, and eggs without the yolk are all healthier sources of protein for people with the metabolic syndrome who are at increased risk for heart disease.

***

The major problem with eating fat is that it is very high in calories (9 calories per gram compared to 4 calories per gram of protein and carbohydrate).

***

Fat is everywhere in our bodies. It lines nerves. It is needed to make normal hormones. And it is a way to store energy. Your muscles use free fatty acids (from fat) for fuel when you are exercising. This is why it is good to exercise for longer than twenty minutes. During the first twenty minutes of exercise your body is burning the readily released stored sugar in your muscles and liver. After twenty minutes, though, you start to break down fat to use for energy.

The major problem with eating fat is that it is very high in calories (9 calories per gram compared to 4 calories per gram of protein and carbohydrate). Unfortunately, it tastes good—especially when it is found in foods such as cookies, cakes, and ice cream. It's okay to eat fat in moderation, but you just need to know which sources of fat are better for you and can help you reduce your risk of heart disease. The two types of fat in food are known as "unsaturated" and "saturated." There are two subcategories of unsaturated fats called "monounsaturated" and "polyunsaturated" fats; these are the ones that help lower your cholesterol level. You can find monounsaturated fats in olive, canola, almond, and peanut oils as well as in avocados. Most other vegetable oils, such as corn, safflower, sunflower, soybean, and cottonseed, are high in polyunsaturated fats. Omega-3 fats are also good for you and may help lower the risk for heart attack and stroke.

Sources of Omega-3 Fats

Cold-water fishes:

Salmon

Herring

Sardines (also a good source of calcium)

Seabass

Haddock

Halibut

Cod

Tuna, canned light

Flounder/sole

Tuna—white albacore or fresh*

Mackerel—king*

Swordfish*

Plant foods:

Flaxseed

Flaxseed oil

Canola oil

Walnuts

Soybeans

Wheat germ

Dried beans

Dark-green leafy vegetables (e.g., spinach, broccoli, kale)

---

*These fish tend to have a higher mercury content than the others, so should be eaten only in moderation.

> **If you see "hydrogenated" or "partially hydrogenated" oils listed as a primary ingredient, beware.**

It is good to lower consumption of saturated fats, which are found mainly in animal products such as meats, whole milk, cheese, butter, lard, shortening, and also in tropical oils such as palm and coconut oil. The way to identify saturated fats is that, like butter, they are solid at room temperature. If you see "hydrogenated" or "partially hydrogenated" oils listed as a primary ingredient, beware. Watch out, too, for the trans-fatty acids (components of trans fats) that are added to processed foods such as cookies and crackers. They are particularly dangerous for people with insulin resistance because they lower the HDL (good) cholesterol and raise the LDL (bad) cholesterol levels. Trans-fatty acids are chemically altered; they are bad for your heart and can lead to weight gain. Effective January 1, 2006, the FDA will be mandating that trans fats be listed on nutrition labels so you can avoid foods that are high in them.

Sources of Trans Fats

French fries and other fried foods

Doughnuts

Store-bought baked goods including pastry, cakes, and cookies

Crackers

Potato chips

Savory snacks

Stick margarines

Some tub margarines

Shortening

Any product that has been "partially hydrogenated"

This table compares the various types of fats—as well as choles-terol, which you recall from chapter 4 also plays an important role in insulin resistance—and their health impact.

I urge you to read food labels. The first thing to look at is how many portions are in the food package. Next, look at what con-stitutes a portion of that particular food. There are times when you may think the calories and carbohydrate grams listed are for the entire container, when in fact they are for only a given amount of it.

Nutrition Facts

Serving Size 1 cup (228g)
Serving Per Container 2   — *portion*

Amount Per Serving

Calories 250   Calories from Fat 110

	% Daily Value*
Total Fat 12g	**18%**
Saturated Fat 3g	**15%**
Cholesterol 30 mg	**10%**
Sodium 470 mg	**20%**
Total Carbohydrate 31g	**10%**
Dietary Fiber 0g	**0%**
Sugars 5g	
Protein 5g	

Vitamin A	4%
Vitamin C	2%
Calcium	20%
Iron	4%

*Percent Daily Values are based on a 2,000 calorie diet. Your Daily Values may be higher or lower depending on your calorie needs:

	Calories	2,000	2,500
Total Fat	Less than	65g	80g
Sat Fat	Less than	20g	25g
Cholesterol	Less than	300mg	300mg
Sodium	Less than	2,400mg	2,400mg
Total Carbohydrate		300g	375g
Dietary Fiber		25g	30g

AN EXAMPLE OF THE NEW FOOD LABEL

TABLE 6

Type of Fat or Cholesterol	Sources	Evaluation
Trans fat	Anything that has been "partially hydrogenated"	Very bad
Saturated fat	Butter, bacon, tropical oils, creamers, chicken and beef fats	Very bad
Cholesterol	Egg yolks, organ meats, cheese, whole milk, veal, lamb, beef	Bad
Polyunsaturated fat	Stick margarine; some tub margarines; mayonnaise; soybean, corn, and safflower oil	OK
Monounsaturated fat	Avocados; pesto sauce; peanut and almond butter; canola, olive, and peanut oil	Good
Omega-3 fats	Fish, flaxseed and canola oils, walnuts (etc.)	Very Good

2. Engage in Daily Physical Activity

Many people make the mistake of starting an exercise program too fast. They jump into an activity, get tired and sore, then decide that it was a bad idea. If you haven't been exercising at all, a better way to start is by doing five to ten minutes of moderate exercise per day and increasing by five to ten minutes each week until you reach forty-five minutes, five times per week. You don't even have to do the activity continuously—exercising in two shorter blocks of time that add up to your target number of minutes is just as good as exercising in one longer block. Choose an activity that you will enjoy. Getting a partner so you can support each other is very effective. Try writing in a date book when, where, and for how long you are going to exercise. You'll be more inclined to keep to your commitment.

You always should ask your physician if it's okay for you to start an exercise program. Your physician undoubtedly will be happy that you want to exercise. But if you have insulin resistance or prediabetes with its increased risk for heart disease, you may need a treadmill test to be sure you can handle the activity. Do not, however, use this an excuse to delay your exercise program. Starting slowly and gradually will allow you to safely increase your intensity over time. Listen to your body, too, for signs of stress, such as chest pain or shortness of breath, which mean you should stop and rest.

3. Learn About Proper Portion Sizes

Sometimes I eat a meal with a patient and I am surprised at how much food they eat, especially since I assume that when they are eating with me they will be on their best behavior. I'm often concerned with their food choices and huge portion sizes. This is particularly true in restaurants where it is normal to have large plates loaded with food. Our super-sized culture has distorted the picture of a normal meal. We all need to consciously retrain ourselves to recognize a reasonable portion size. A rough count of calories and carbohydrates can stop you from eating excessive amounts of food at each meal.

***Our super-sized culture has distorted
the picture of a normal meal.***

TABLE 7. COMMON PORTION SIZES

Measurement	Visual Reference	Calories and Carbohydrates
Starch: ½ cup (pasta, cooked cereal) (except rice, where ⅓ cup is a portion size)	Palm of your hand for ½ cup; less than that for ⅓ cup	60–90 calories 15 grams of carbohydrate
Fruit: 1 piece (small to medium size)	Fits easily into the palm of your hand— about the size of a tennis ball	60–90 calories 15 grams of carbohydrate
Vegetables (except starchy veggies like peas, lima beans, and corn): 2–3 cups; in many cases unlimited	Should fill up half of your plate	0–50 calories 10–15 grams of carbohydrate
Milk: 8 ounces	One small glass— check to see if the glass holds 8 ounces	60–90 calories 12 grams of carbohydrate
Protein: 3 ounces	Should fit into the palm of your hand— about the size of a deck of cards	35–100 calories no carbohydrate
Fat: 1 teaspoon (This includes cooking oils as well as salad dressings and gravies. Try to avoid saturated and trans fats)	Hold your thumb up— from the tip of your thumb down to the first joint is one teaspoon	45 calories no carbohydrate

The other behavior I've noticed when dining with my patients is that they clean their plates down to every last morsel of food. This is true even when they don't seem to like the food they are eating all that much. After the point when their hunger is satisfied they still seem to feel bound to eat everything served.

During college I had access to unlimited supplies of high-carbohydrate and high-fat food in our dining hall. The freedom of unlimited good food led to my gaining about 20 extra pounds. So I started reading books on how to lose the excess weight. I ended up following an Atkins-type diet over a summer break and lost the weight I had gained. It was easy to follow because my food choices (and student budget) were so limited. Afterward, I wanted to make sure I kept the weight off. So I started to study the habits of thin people (a study I continue to this day). What stuck with me is that thin people never cleaned their plate. I started to make this a habit and to this day I still consciously leave some food uneaten. I eat consciously, always with a voice in my head that says "stop" once I have eaten enough. So far, it's worked for me and I think it can work for you.

4. Use the Plate Method to Balance Meals and Control Portions

After you have learned portion sizes, try to put together a healthy meal in your mind. To do this, visualize a 9-inch dinner plate or get some 9-inch paper plates to use for props. Don't use an oversized plate (tableware, like portion size, has also become bigger over the years). Half of the meal you visualize on your plate should be vegetables and/or salad. The other half is divided in half again, with one part devoted to protein (3 to 4 ounces) and the other part to carbohydrates (1 cup). Now, try this same exercise using real food

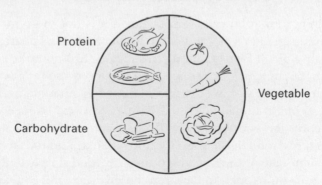

ED'S THREE-PORTION SPECIAL

at home. You can play with the food a bit, measuring out portions, comparing them to your own "fist measure," then dumping the food out on your plate. This practice will help you estimate portion size when you eat in restaurants.

My nutritionist, Meg, has a blind patient named Ed who likes eating out. Ed decided to simply describe the plate method to the waiter every time he ordered a meal, giving the waiter a very clear and quite visual idea of what he wanted to eat. With a little practice Ed usually got what he wanted—and he lost 10 pounds in six weeks.

5. Keep Food Consumption Records

The conscious act of writing down everything you eat is a surprisingly effective weight loss technique. Logging your food intake within fifteen minutes of eating helps you be aware of how many calories you consume and allows you to discover opportunities to change your patterns. The log shows what you are doing well and highlights where you can improve. For example, you may find that you have not had any vegetables for the past five days. I know that my twelve-year-old son would prefer never to see vegetables in his diet, except for French fries (which hardly count as a vegetable). Just as I have to encourage my son to eat healthier foods, you need to encourage yourself to eat correctly by objectively looking at what you need to add or subtract from your diet.

6. Clean Up Your Food Environment

Like a siren, junk food calls to you. But if it is not there in your pantry or refrigerator, you can't eat it. In the weight loss phase, you don't want difficult foods around. This means throw out the cookies, candy, potato chips, ice cream, and whatever else tempts you. In America we seem to have this fear of throwing out food, perhaps because so many adults today had parents who experienced the Great Depression and World War II rationing. Frankly, it is much better to throw food in the trash than to add extra pounds to your body. I am not advocating buying unhealthy food simply to throw it out. But if you happen to have purchased chips or ice cream to feed to guests, throw the extra out rather than eating it yourself. It would be great if we could safely repackage excess food and send it to people who are hungry, but it's not good for them either! So get rid of it (and not by eating it).

In America we seem to have this fear of throwing out food, perhaps because so many adults today had parents who experienced the Great Depression and World War II rationing.

Limiting access does help. I have had several nannies for my son who came from small Midwestern towns. When they first arrived at my house they were surprised that we didn't have a junk food drawer. They were equally surprised by the variety of fresh fruits and vegetables available. And although I didn't limit the food they purchased, they tended to eat as we did. Most lost weight as a result.

7. Learn to Know Your Hunger

Knowing your hunger is knowing the difference between physical and emotional hunger. Learn to determine if you are really hungry by being conscious of when you last ate. Ask yourself (and answer honestly) if you are physically hungry or are actually lonely, bored, or depressed. If you feel hungry and have eaten a balanced meal within the past two hours, for instance, you are probably suffering more from emotional than physical hunger. Late-night snacking usually fills an emotional need for companionship or entertain-ment or as a release from the stress of the day, the job, and/or the family. It's better to identify when you are vulnerable to emotional eating and to develop strategies, in advance, to deal with it. If you have a tendency to eat late in the evening, do something else instead. Walk on a treadmill or work out on an Exercycle, or eat food that is low in calories and high in fiber (such as raw vegetables or fruit).

It's better to identify when you are vulnerable to emotional eating and to develop strategies, in advance, to deal with it.

Be smart about choosing snacks. Buying raw peanuts in the shell makes you open and eat them one at a time. Such snacks limit your ability to consume them in bulk, and you eat them slowly enough so that the physiological signals of being full can enter into your consciousness and help control the emotional need to eat. There can be occasions where you will indulge emotional eating, but you must learn to forgive yourself as quickly as possible. The next day can and will be better. You don't have to give in to a self-fulfilling negative prophecy of overeating, self-loathing, and despair, which only leads to more overeating.

8. Eat and Drink Small Amounts Often, So You Never Feel Too Hungry

Eat three meals and two snacks each day. The best meals are combinations of fat, carbohydrate, and protein. Ideally you should keep your carbohydrate intake to less than 40 percent of your total calories. This generally means eating 60 grams of carbohydrate or less per meal. You can learn to measure this by looking at food labels and buying a carbohydrate counting guide.

An easy way to limit carbohydrates is to avoid food that is white. For instance, brown rice is better than white rice, and brown whole grain bread is better than white bread. The more cooked or mashed a food is, the more quickly its sugar is absorbed, creating more stress on your body. A whole, fresh apple with the skin is better than a baked apple, which in turn is better than applesauce. Food that is higher in fiber and less processed tends to be absorbed more slowly. It stays around in your digestive track longer, producing a sense of fullness. In addition, when carbohydrate is taken up quickly into your bloodstream insulin is released rapidly, and I personally believe that this rapid rise and fall of insulin makes you feel hungry sooner. It also may make you feel more tired after eating. Remember, we were never, ever meant to drink sugar as a liquid. Fruit juices and sodas are a man-made invention and not what our intestines evolved to handle.

**An easy way to limit carbohydrates
is to avoid food that is white.**

The glycemic index is a chart that tells you how rapidly carbohydrate is absorbed as sugar into your bloodstream compared to either drinking sugar water or eating a piece of white bread. The lower the glycemic index, the slower the food is absorbed. Food like lentils have a very low glycemic index because they are absorbed as sugar very slowly due to their high natural fiber content (see pp. 169–170).

Scientists have gone back and forth debating whether or not the glycemic index is valid. Based on my clinical experience with people and the foods they eat I know that certain carbohydrates are absorbed much more quickly and have a different effect on how a person feels than other forms of carbohydrate. Therefore, no matter what the science is, you have to learn to listen to your own body. This means that it is important to know yourself and to identify which foods make you feel full for a long time, which foods seem to make you tired, or which ones just leave you craving more to eat after only an hour or two.

Snacks should be small and relatively filling, and should follow the model of combining food from all three types of foods. A handful of trail mix is a good snack, as is half an apple with peanut butter, or a few sticks of celery filled with low-fat cream cheese, or a stick of string cheese.

**No matter what the science is, you have
to learn to listen to your own body.**

Protein should come from sources that are low in saturated fat—turkey, chicken, fish, and soy are excellent sources of protein. If you like to eat red meat, choose cuts that are as lean as possible. I have seen way too many pictures of arteries filled with plaque to think that eating bacon every day is good for you. However, an occasional egg (particularly if you make omelets out of a mixture of whole eggs plus egg whites) is okay.

Finally, drink water. We recommend 64 ounces of water daily. It's fine to mix in other liquids with water; you can drink decaffeinated coffee, tea, or calorie-free drinks to help you meet this goal (but don't go overboard on diet sodas, especially those with caffeine). Drinking this much fluid will increase how much you urinate and it is wise not to drink a lot in the hours before bedtime. There is no magic to drinking fluids, except that they help you feel full and allow you to put something in your mouth without taking in calories. If you can lose weight without drinking so many fluids, that's fine. Unless you are very old or have had a stroke, your body will tell you when it is thirsty.

There is no magic to drinking fluids, except that they help you feel full and allow you to put something in your mouth without taking in calories.

---

9. Don't Be a Slave to the Scale

Weigh yourself once a week. Establish a routine—time of day, clothes to wear (or not wear). Be sure your scale is on a flat surface and calibrates to zero. If you have had a week of eating wisely don't get discouraged if you haven't lost any weight. Weight loss is slow and your goal is to establish new habits that allow you to gradually lose weight and be healthier. It is not a race to have some sudden, extraordinary weight loss. Remember, it took a while to gain the weight. And sometimes, it's how you look and feel, not what you weigh, that counts.

10. Plan Your Meals for a Week at a Time

Here are some ideas that can help you save time for enjoying other activities (hint: such as exercise):

- Limit your grocery shopping to once a week. The more often you go to the store, the more tempted you are to buy extra items you just do not need.

- Clean and chop up your fruits and vegetables in advance, for easy access. Keep them in sealed plastic bags or containers in your refrigerator. That way, they will be staring you in the face when you're rummaging around looking for food. And once you've spent the time chopping them up, you may be motivated not to let them go to waste and will eat them instead of less healthy choices.

- Buy skinned and boneless chicken for easy preparation.

- Keep staples in the house to make a quick healthy meal. If you dislike cooking, you can always double the recipe and freeze half for later use.

- Learn to read labels. If you tend to heat premade meals instead of cooking, the labels can help you meet the target of less than 60 grams of carbohydrates per meal.

Most thin people work at being thin—it just doesn't come naturally in today's excessive food environment.

---

11. Eat More Fruits and Vegetables

We recommend two servings of fruit and three of vegetables every day. This may be impossible for you to achieve on a daily basis, but if you are conscious about increasing your intake, it will help. Take, for example, a buffet of appetizers at a dinner party. Often there will be hot appetizers and crackers and cheese and then a tray or two of cut celery, carrots, and other raw vegetables. If you gravitate toward the latter, you will increase your vegetable consumption and decrease the calorie total. On that little buffet plate you can easily load 600 to 800 calories in cheese, crackers, and hot appetizers. When I go out to lunch or dinner with some of my ultrathin, very fashion conscious friends, I realize that they don't eat "normally" to stay thin. Even in the fanciest restaurants they order salads or vegetables, dishes like non-cream based soup, or entrées without sauces. Most thin people work at being thin—it just doesn't come naturally in today's excessive food environment.

Meg once had a patient named Cathy, who gained weight on the Atkin's diet because she was consuming mostly high-fat protein foods such as cheese, bacon, and red meat. Meg added more carbohydrates to Cathy's diet, such as whole grain bread, beans, fruit, low-fat milk, and vegetables, while advising her to avoid some of the refined carbohydrates, such as pasta, light bread, and rice because they don't provide as much nutritional value and fiber. On this diet, Cathy was able to lose the weight that she couldn't on Atkin's.

12. If You Smoke, Quit!

Most people think of smoking in terms of increasing the risk for cancer, but it also increases the risk for heart attack and stroke, particularly if you have insulin resistance. When I have a patient who has prediabetes or diabetes who smokes, I discuss smoking cessation at every visit until they stop.

Methods to quit smoking are varied, and most of the people I know who have stopped successfully seem to do it cold turkey, rather than by tapering down. Nicotine patches and gums are readily available, and I have found Zyban (which is really the antidepressant known as Wellbutrin) quite helpful. I usually start patients out on low doses of Wellbutrin, maybe 100 milligrams per day, and gradually work them up to 150 mg twice per day, which is the full dose of Zyban. Many different programs and support groups exist to help people stop smoking. We in the medical profession really want you to quit, so ask your health care provider for recommendations.

....

*"Find something else that you love
to replace the food you give up."*

Putting all of these pieces together sounds simple on paper, but I know that it's more difficult to put into practice in real life. I have made these points thousands of times to patients, but never really understood what I was asking until my husband was diagnosed with prediabetes. I suddenly saw firsthand the challenges and frustrations that occur when a health care professional says, "Change your lifestyle and follow these new patterns." I also learned how much these lifestyle changes can help improve health. Here is Mark's story.

Food was never that much of an issue for me. At least not eating too much food. I didn't like all the shopping, cooking, and cleaning up. I actively look forward to those science fiction days where I'm able to satisfy my hunger with a food pill.

I never suspected that I had prediabetes. Sure I was a little tired mid-mornings, but who thought that it was related to that big bowl of cereal with sliced banana I ate every morning? Anne gave me a glucose meter and made me stab my finger three to four times a day. I thought it was a useless exercise, but we were newly in love and I put up with the pain.

I was tall, lean, and looked nothing like the Homer Simpson cartoon that she showed at her talks as an example of the diabetic shape. But even when I was quite active, I could never seem to get my belly to have that six-pack, cut look. No matter how many sit-ups I did there still was a bit of a bulge. And as I got older, I wasn't playing volleyball or tennis as often as I once was.

My blood sugar numbers came back high. They were around 110 before breakfast and went up to 180 to 210 after eating. There was no doubt I had prediabetes. Anne set me up with her nutritionist to talk about my diet. I learned about the concept of limiting my meals to 60 grams of carbohydrates. I had to start paying attention to food labels and had to give up my cereal and my beloved chicken burritos.

I increased my exercise. Mostly I walked on our treadmill while watching TV in the evenings, but I also came out of volleyball retirement. I don't worry about being a serious weekend warrior anymore. I just play for the fun and exercise now.

The change in my diet at first made it harder to find foods to eat. I won't make many fans by telling you that this shift in eating habits caused me to lose 20 pounds quite effortlessly. Some of it has come back, but I still find controlling my weight easy. My blood sugars came down, but according to my doctor, not quite enough. So she put me on Actos, a pill that decreases insulin resistance, and that did the trick.

I would go to talks with Anne and she would embarrass me by having me stand as she told my story. I would tell this group of doctors at the dinner gathering that my secret was switching from drinking beer to wine. This is a simplified truth about preventing diabetes. Find something else that you love to replace the food you give up. My favorite hearty amber ales carried a load of 40 grams of carbs a bottle. A glass of merlot has zero carbs. This food substitution business wasn't all that hard after all.

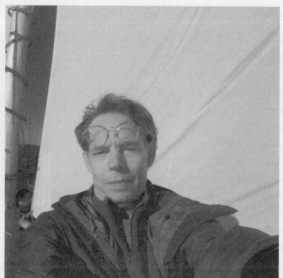

Breakfast is now a carton of yogurt and a food bar with my cup of coffee. The glucose meter is back to being one of my photo props and I exercise enough to cheat on my 60-gram carb limit from time to time. But I still take special care of my heart by taking a low-dose adult aspirin and Zetia to lower my cholesterol. I know more about diabetes than I ever wanted, but I don't consider it a burden. I'm just paying attention to my body's needs and choosing to be healthy. And I have my doctor wife to bug me if I don't take care of myself.

....

DIET FOR CARBOHYDRATE-SENSITIVE HYPOGLYCEMIA

Carbohydrate-sensitive hypoglycemia is described as feeling hungry, shaky, and sweaty one to three hours after eating carbohydrates. Treatment is to follow a lower carbohydrate diet, similar to that used for treating all types of insulin resistance. You want to be sure not to eat too much carbohydrate anyway, particularly not simple carbohydrate, at any one time. That's why we recommend that you have at least three meals and two snacks each day. Some people even have three snacks each day. Most simple carbohydrates, such as fruit juices, jellies, jams, syrup, regular soda, pure sugar, and honey should be avoided if you have reactive hypoglycemia due to the increase of insulin response. The goal is to have the carbohydrate intake between 40 and 45 percent of total calories, protein between 15 and 20 percent of total calories, and fat between 30 and 35 percent of total calories.

Try to spread your carbohydrates evenly throughout the day. If you are eating 1,500 calories and you want to have a 40 percent carbohydrate diet, you would have 150 grams of carbs per day. This translates to 30 grams for breakfast, 15 for snack, 45 for lunch, 15 for snack, and 45 for dinner. In food terms you would be having, for example, an egg with sautéed vegetables and two slices of whole grain toast or a whole wheat English muffin for breakfast. A snack could be ½ cup of cottage cheese and a piece of cut-up fruit. Lunch could be salad with grilled chicken and black beans with a whole grain roll and margarine. The midday snack could be cheese and four crackers. Then dinner would be grilled fish, lots of green veggies, salad, ⅔ cup of brown rice, and 1 cup of berries with whipped cream. Doesn't sound so bad, does it?

Tips for Reducing Carbohydrate-Sensitive Hypoglycemia

- Spread your carbohydrates throughout the day.

- Avoid simple sugars, such as candy, juice, and regular soda, especially between meals.

- Increase fiber-rich foods, such as beans, whole wheat products, veggies, and fruits. Fresh fruit always is preferred to fruit juices.

- Include some protein and fat in all your meals and snacks. Mixed food groups are best.

EXERCISE IN THE TREATMENT OF PREDIABETES

Although exercise without weight loss does not prevent diabetes, it has many benefits in terms of improving sensitivity to insulin and lowering the risk for heart disease. Many patients ask if they absolutely have to exercise. The answer is, unequivocally, yes. If you wish to maintain maximal levels of health, the best approach to exercise includes both aerobic exercise and resistance training.

The benefits to exercise include the following:

- Increased strength and endurance

- Improved circulation

- Improved bone health

- Decreased stress

- Improved insulin sensitivity

- Improved glucose tolerance

- Lower rates of osteoporosis (thinning of the bones)

- Fewer and less damaging falls (a common problem in the elderly)

- Improved joint strength and mobility

- Lower rates of heart disease

- Lower rates of cancer

- Lower rates of depression (which can lead to emotional eating)

In most cases, we create our own barriers, obstacles, and excuses.

If you have questions about your overall fitness, check with your doctor before you start an exercise program to obtain the go-ahead to proceed. It may actually be more important to check with your doctor before *stopping* your exercise. Choose an activity that you will enjoy. Some options are walking, bicycling, swimming, dancing, jumping rope, cross-country skiing, skating, Pilates, and water aerobics. After you find what type of exercise is best suited to you, you should choose a time of day in which you will exercise.

This should be kept consistent. Treat it as an appointment with yourself to exercise. It must be a time that you honor each day— your exercise time. Establish a routine. Start slowly if you have not been working out. Don't worry if you exercise only for five minutes at a time in the beginning. You always can increase the minutes as your energy improves.

Be aware that situations may arise that can cause you to get off track from your exercise program. Illness, holidays, vacations, child care, or work conflicts will come up. Instead of being discouraged and giving up, create an alternative plan that can accommodate all of your schedules and lifestyle. In most cases, we create our own barriers, obstacles, and excuses. So, with a little planning you can stay on track and be successful. For instance, a patient of mine told me that he was great at exercising when he was at home, but couldn't do it when he was on the road. I mentioned that I routinely use the gym in hotels when I travel. He countered with the excuse that since he was a recognizable celebrity, people came up to him and talked to him when he worked out in a public area, and that made him uncomfortable. The solution was to have the hotel put an Exercycle in his room when he arrived, so he could continue his morning exercise habit undisturbed. Doing this has helped him stick to his exercise regimen consistently, with measurable benefits to his health. Granted, he may have gotten preferential treatment because of his celebrity status and could afford to stay in hotels with such amenities. But with a little ingenuity anyone can maintain an exercise schedule while traveling.

Stretching and weight training also help you to burn fat and sugar more efficiently when you do exercise.

You should strive to exercise forty-five to sixty minutes per day for five days each week. Although this sounds like a lot when you are first starting out, before you know it you will not notice the time going by. I choose to watch TV when I exercise, generally a show that runs for an hour. It tends to be the only television I watch each night, but linking it to exercise helps me stick to my exercise commitment—not to mention keep up on my TV viewing.

When you exercise, remember to warm up before to prevent injuries and cool down afterward to slow your breathing. Along with raising your heart rate during exercise, it is important to strengthen and stretch your muscles. Making your muscles stronger helps to prevent injuries and helps you to be more physically independent as you grow older. Stretching and weight training also help you to burn fat and sugar more efficiently when you do exercise. Diabetes can cause some stiffening of the muscles, as can aging and the exercise itself. So be sure to stretch your muscles every time you work out. Always warm up your muscles, too, by walking around a bit before you stretch them. Stretching muscles when they are cold (meaning that you've been sitting still and not moving around at all) could cause pulls or nagging injuries.

Warming up may be less important at first, when you aren't exercising much, but as you gradually increase your exercise intensity this will become more helpful. Therefore, you should start with good habits from the beginning and incorporate a five-minute warm-up prior to each exercise session. Increase your exercise gradually, in slow increments until you are doing thirty to forty-five minutes per day of aerobic exercise (exercise that increases your heart rate and usually involves brisk movement). In addition, try to incorporate ten to twenty minutes of weight training, using three- to five-pound weights and gentle strengthening exercises. You don't want to do anything too hard or too intensive at first. Injuries could set you back. Your body will tell you the exercise level that is best for you.

Some people have a target heart rate for maximal fitness. The problem with these targets is that many people are not able to reach and maintain these targets due to health issues or medications. Do these people still get health benefits from exercise? Absolutely! Any exercise is good exercise.

If you want to know your target heart rate get out your calculators and use the following formula. Subtract your age from 220, then multiply that result by 0.7. For a fifty-year-old this works out as $220 - 50 = 170$. And $170 \times 0.7 = 119$. Therefore, this patient should attempt to increase his heart rate to 119 while exercising and maintain that pulse for at least thirty minutes. A heart rate monitor also can be used to give you continuous feedback and allow you to skip the math.

TABLE 8. ESTIMATED NUMBER OF CALORIES BURNED DURING VARIOUS ACTIVITIES

These values are only approximate—intensity of exercise, weight, and body composition all change the calories burned. Exercise machines often allow for entry of body weight and will estimate calories expended per hour as well as per exercise session.

Type of Activity	Calories Used per Hour (150-pound person)	Calories Used per Hour (200-pound person)
Bicycling (14 to 16 mph)	720	960
Bicycling (stationary)	504	672
Bowling	216	288
Gardening	324	432
Golf (carrying clubs)	396	528
Golf (riding in golf cart)	252	336
Raking lawn	288	384
Running (8 minutes per mile)	900	1200
Running (12 minutes per mile)	576	768
Sitting (reading, watching TV)	81	108
Sleeping	45	60
Swimming	432	576
Tennis	504	672
Walking (13 minutes per mile)	360	480

How Can We Tempt You to Exercise?

Patients with diabetes often ask, "What type of exercise should I do?" My reply is to find activities you like, ones that you look forward to each day and that can be done in some form or another for the rest of your life. Rotate activities so your exercise routine won't get boring or stale. The way you exercise may change as you age—it is the exercise habit that should remain consistent. Someone who has not been exercising is bound to say to me, "Well, I don't love any type of exercise. I hate exercise." I try to help these patients find something that can make exercise fun. If someone likes listening to music I suggest they listen to their favorite music when they work out. Or I suggest that patients find an interesting or beautiful place where they can exercise and think about nature. Getting a dog is a good (and persistent) way to be motivated to go out walking. If patients enjoy groups, I suggest going to local classes at a health club, Curves, YMCA, or community center. Sometimes it helps to find a partner to exercise with, such as a friend, spouse, or coworker. However, getting exercise cannot solely be dependent on another person for motivation, because you still need to exercise if your partner is not around.

Getting a dog is a good (and persistent) way to be motivated to go out walking.

If nothing discussed above seems to make any difference, I ask patients about sports. Sometimes I can coax out the old competitive college or high school athlete inside them, and use that for motivation. People may like exercising with their kids. I ask patients what their children like to do and see if there is a way for the family to go hiking, biking, or in-line skating together (with appropriate protective gear). Sometimes I try to probe more deeply and ask, "What did you do when you were a kid? What kind of activities did you like?" Often people respond, "I am too old to exercise." I won't take that as an excuse. I explain that people who are older can derive the same benefits from exercise as younger people. If anything, older people need to exercise more. The

YMCA has great programs for seniors, including an interactive program called Twinges and Hinges for people with arthritis who can't exercise in standard exercise classes.

STRESS AND PREDIABETES

Intense stress can increase blood sugar levels in individuals without the diagnosis of diabetes. Severe stress during a serious illness is accompanied by an increase in hormones called "counterregulatory" hormones. They are designed to make sure you have plenty of sugar in your bloodstream to help you react to intense situations. These hormones cause the liver to release sugar and to make the body more resistant to the effects of insulin, which would lower blood sugar levels.

Although stress by itself will not cause prediabetes in someone who is not at risk, it can affect our behaviors and blood sugar levels in a variety of ways. Therefore, it is useful to try to reduce the stress in your life. Try to identify the situations that cause you stress; it can help to create a log of these things, so you can work on ways to reduce or eliminate the stress. It also helps to note how you respond to stress. Some stressed-out people turn to food, others feel exhausted and go to bed, others feel overwhelmed and have trouble following their lifestyle plan. In the Diabetes Prevention Program it helped many participants to talk with a social worker and deal with reducing some of their life stressors so they could see clear to change their diet and exercise patterns.

Try to identify the situations that cause you stress; it can help to create a log of these things, so you can work on ways to reduce or eliminate the stress.

The following is a list of ideas that can help you deal with stress:

- Practice deep breathing.
- Incorporate yoga into your life (a very helpful accompaniment to an exercise program).

- Meditate.

- Get a massage.

- Encourage yourself to have positive thoughts and reduce the number of negative thoughts you allow. (For example, when I do public presentations and am backstage waiting to speak, I push out all thoughts that are negative and self-doubting. I allow only positive thoughts in and visualize myself being successful. I guarantee you will do a better job than if you let your head fill with thoughts of insecurity and inadequacy.)

- Take a bath. (Go ahead, pamper yourself—use bubble bath and candles, play music. Let yourself fully relax for a little while.)

- Avoid fatty or spicy foods.

- Listen to music.

- Read a book that really interests you—whether fiction or nonfiction. Or try some poetry.

- Learn to say no if you are being overwhelmed with tasks. If you can't say no, then learn to delegate.

- Keep a journal. Write down your thoughts and feelings.

Lifestyle changes are probably the most powerful tools we have for preventing type 2 diabetes. Recent undesirable changes in lifestyle, with an increase in caloric intake and a decrease in physical activity, have led to the current diabetes epidemic. Unfortunately, changing lifestyle is hard. Most of us rebel or try to do it for a while, but then revert to our old habits. With prediabetes and diabetes, however, changing lifestyle can make a big difference. It just has to be done with help, with a health care team that can make recommendations that will fit your life. I've watched patient after patient, including my husband Mark, change diet and exercise habits in order to prevent getting diabetes. And it works! Healthier habits in conjunction with some of the medications we now have can significantly lower your risk of diabetes and heart disease. Long-term health is a goal worth fighting for.

EIGHT

BEYOND LIFESTYLE CHANGES: MEDICATIONS THAT TREAT PREDIABETES

We think that certain drugs can help prevent diabetes. The final verdict isn't in yet, but as I'll explain, we have strong signals that these new medications work.[6] We do, however, know for sure that there are drugs that can lower your risk of heart attack and stroke (such as those that lower blood pressure, cholesterol, and triglycerides, and reduce your risk of blood clots). Though I'm going to tell you about several different medications that can help people with prediabetes, I also want to be clear that there is nothing more important for your health than to eat well and exercise on a regular basis. All of the medications work best when they are combined with changes of lifestyle. If there is enough of a change, medication may not be needed at all.

I don't like pills much myself, but I take them when I need to.

I tend to see patients I can roughly classify in two groups. The first group just wants a pill or two (or ten) to fix whatever is wrong with them. They don't want to change their habits and don't mind taking medication. The second group hates taking pills because of potential adverse reactions and a dislike of putting chemicals into their bodies. I don't like pills much myself, but I take them when I need to. What I try to make clear to my patients is that we are trying to achieve a balance between lifestyle changes and taking appropriate medication. Some patients need to take many different pills. The average person with diabetes takes nine different pills each day to prevent complications. This breaks down to two to three pills for lowering blood sugar, two to three for lowering blood pressure, one to two for treatment of abnormal cholesterol and triglyceride levels, and an aspirin to lower the risk for blood clotting. But whenever you take medication you should always know how it works, the potential side effects, how it might interact with other medications, and how to monitor the drugs and their effects on your body. I check every medication my patients take. I do it at each subsequent visit. I am the pill police.

WHAT YOU NEED TO KNOW ABOUT ANY MEDICATION

- How it works

- When you should take it and whether or not you can take it with food or other medication

- The potential side effects

- How it may interact with other medications

- What monitoring is required, if any, for its continued use

It is vital that you keep track of your medications and ask your physician specifically about interactions. Sometimes your pharmacist can be helpful in this regard, as long as you get all of your medications from the same place. I have found people taking not only the wrong pills for simultaneously existing conditions, but often the right pills in incorrect doses. Consequently, I try to write down a daily schedule for each patient and explain exactly which pills should be taken at what time of day.

THE DIABETES PREVENTION PROGRAM, PART 2: MEDICATIONS

You'll recall the Diabetes Prevention Program (DPP) study from chapter 7. In essence, it was a study designed to test the benefits of three different therapies on the prevention of diabetes in patients at high risk for developing the disease: diet and exercise; metformin, which lowers production of sugar from the liver; and troglitazone, which decreases insulin resistance. The study included a control or placebo group, which entailed no special treatment. The participants all had impaired glucose tolerance, or increases in their blood sugar levels above the normal range, but were below the level necessary to diagnose diabetes. The study showed that losing 15 pounds and exercising five days a week for thirty minutes at a time was effective in preventing diabetes. But this study also showed that medication can help.

The use of the medications in this study was experimental. The drugs used had been approved by the FDA for the treatment of diabetes, but not approved for diabetes prevention. This doesn't mean that the study drugs are unsafe to use in the prevention of diabetes. It just means that they haven't been extensively studied for preventative purposes, and therefore most insurance companies won't pay for this use. Moreover, not all doctors agree on using these drugs to prevent diabetes. In certain circumstances I will use them, and I'll tell you why. It's perfectly understandable to be hesitant about using medication to prevent diabetes. I still believe that weight loss and exercise are the two best treatments we have for diabetes prevention. But if those aren't working well enough, then medication should be considered.

There currently are several large studies under way to determine whether medication truly is useful for the prevention of diabetes in both adolescents and adults. Within a few years we will have more data from these trials. Chapter 11 discusses the use of oral diabetes medications in detail.

Drugs That May Help Prevent Diabetes

- Metformin (Glucophage)

- Glitazones: pioglitazone (Actos); rosiglitazone (Avandia) (The original drug in this class, troglitazone [Rezulin], was pulled from the market.)

- Alpha-glucosidase inhibitors: acarbose (Precose); miglitol (Glyset)

Metformin

Metformin has been used worldwide in the treatment of diabetes since 1957. (I discuss it in more detail in chapter 11 in relation to the treatment of type 2 diabetes.) Metformin is the drug's generic name; it is sold under the trade names of Glucophage and Glucophage XR in the United States. Approximately one thousand patients in the DPP study took metformin. They lowered their risk of getting diabetes by about one-third and had a slight weight loss (about 3 pounds) as compared to the control group. There were no serious side effects from the metformin. Patients do need to be carefully selected before starting this drug, and should have a normal kidney function as determined by a blood test for creatinine level—test results must show levels less than 1.4 mg/dl in females and less than 1.5 mg/dl in males. If you have congestive heart failure, significant liver damage, or other serious medical conditions, you should not be on metformin. Ask your doctor if metformin is safe for you, or review the patient package insert.

Metformin is a very good drug for the treatment of actual diabetes, but for some reason (perhaps because it doesn't directly reduce insulin resistance) it did not prevent diabetes in many patients in the DPP. Patients with a normal body weight or who were older than forty-five didn't see much benefit from it. But if you are in your twenties or thirties, are overweight, and are at risk for getting diabetes (particularly if your blood sugar levels are going up), metformin may help prevent diabetes or effectively treat early diabetes. Once someone gets diabetes, metformin may be very effective, especially in the early stages, before blood sugar levels are very high. If blood sugars are seriously elevated, metformin might have less effect.

The Glitazones: A Bumpy Start for a Good Class of Drugs

The thiazolidinediones (TZDs or glitazones, for short) are the newest class of drugs available for the treatment of diabetes. From all the data we have on these drugs, they look to be the best oral medication for preventing diabetes. We still need more data to be sure, but my hunch is that they will turn out to be quite effective for diabetes prevention.

The first drug in this class to come on the market (1996) was troglitazone (Rezulin). Glitazones work by decreasing insulin resistance, making the body more sensitive to insulin and reversing one of the most basic defects in diabetes. The improvements in insulin sensitivity are similar to those from weight loss and exercise. The investigators planning the DPP liked the benefits enough to include troglitazone as an arm in their diabetes prevention study, even though it was not yet on the market for use in the treatment of diabetes. This decision initially made scientific sense, although what was not widely appreciated at the time was the potential for troglitazone to cause severe and even fatal liver damage.

The study results showed that troglitazone lowered the risk for getting diabetes by 73 percent.

One of the study subjects in the DPP had a rare liver reaction to the troglitazone and died. This was incredibly unfortunate, primarily for the patient and her family, and secondarily for science. Troglitazone was part of the DPP study for only ten months. But in the results from the first year, it was the most effective approach to lowering insulin resistance and, thus, for the prevention of diabetes. The study results showed that troglitazone lowered the risk for getting diabetes by 73 percent. Unfortunately we can't draw any firm conclusions from the use of troglitazone in the DPP trial because the use of the drug was stopped too early. The results do suggest, however, that drugs in the same family as troglitazone can prevent the development of type 2 diabetes.

Another, smaller study was done to look at the benefits of troglitazone in the prevention of type 2 diabetes. This trial was called the TRIPOD (*T*roglitazone *i*n the *P*revention *o*f *D*iabetes) study and was done by one of my colleagues at USC, Dr. Tom Buchanan. He studied women who had had gestational diabetes and had a very high risk for getting diabetes in the next five years. They all had impaired glucose tolerance. None were pregnant or planning on becoming pregnant. All were overweight Latino women in their thirties. Dr. Buchanan randomized them (by flipping a coin) to take either troglitazone or a placebo pill. He planned to follow them for many years, but had to stop the study after two and a half years because troglitazone was pulled off the US market.

His preliminary results showed that the troglitazone meaningfully reduced the risk for developing type 2 diabetes in the women who took it. The reduction in risk for getting diabetes with the troglitazone was almost identical to that seen with the diet and exercise therapy in the DPP. We can't use troglitazone anymore, but now there are relatives of troglitazone on the market: pioglitazone and rosiglitazone. These drugs seem much safer than troglitazone. So Dr. Buchanan has restarted his study as PIPOD (*P*ioglitazone *i*n the *P*revention *o*f *D*iabetes) and has begun treating all of his patients from the TRIPOD study with pioglitazone. His first year of using pioglitazone is showing similar results to the risk reduction he found with troglitazone. So the new pioglitazone and rosiglitazone are also probably effective in the prevention of diabetes.

Alpha-Glucosidase Inhibitors: Small Benefits and Annoying Side Effects

Another medication option is alpha-glucosidase inhibitors (AGIs). There are two on the market, acarbose (Precose) and miglitol (Glyset). In theory, these drugs seem as if they would be useful in the prevention and treatment of diabetes. What they do is limit the amount of glucose that is absorbed after a meal. They stay in the intestine and bind starches to prevent their release into the bloodstream. The problem with these drugs is if the starch isn't absorbed in the small intestine, it goes on to the bacteria-rich large intestine. These bacteria break down carbohydrate by fermenting it. Unfortunately, a major by-product of fermentation is gas (like bubbles in beer). This causes patients to have lots of gas and flatulence—uncomfortable and potentially embarrassing—when they take these drugs. AGIs also aren't particularly effective and cause only a very small lowering of blood glucose levels.

In spite of all of these problems, when studied in patients at risk for getting diabetes the alpha-glucosidase inhibitors reduced the risk for developing diabetes by about 25 percent in the diabetes prevention study called STOP-NIDDM. This reduction was much less than that found with diet and exercise and troglitazone or metformin, but it was still meaningful. Even a slight lowering in blood sugar levels after eating can lead to lowering of the risk for getting type 2 diabetes, but I personally have never prescribed AGIs for diabetes prevention.

MEDICATIONS TO LOWER THE RISK OF HEART ATTACK AND STROKE IN PATIENTS WITH PREDIABETES AND THE METABOLIC SYNDROME

Lowering the risk for heart disease and stroke (macrovascular disease) in patients who are at risk for developing diabetes is at least as important as lowering blood sugar levels. There are three treatment goals:

- Lower bad cholesterol levels and raise good cholesterol levels.

- Lower blood pressure (which often is increased in patients at risk for diabetes).

- Lower the tendency of the blood to clot and form life-threatening plaque in arteries.

In many ways treating these problems is simple. Diet and exercise helps them all. However, other simple measures also can help lower risk. The chief medications are listed here.

Drugs to Lower Cholesterol Levels

- Statins, such as pravastatin (Pravachol), fluvastatin (Lescol), lovastatin (Mevacor), simvastatin (Zocor), atorvastatin (Lipitor), rosuvastatin (Crestor)

- Ezetimibe (Zetia)

Drugs to Lower Triglyceride Levels

• Fibric acid derivatives, such as gemfibrozil (Lopid), fenofibrate (Tricor)

• Niacin (Niaspan)

Drugs to Lower Blood Pressure (see pages 232–233 for complete list)

• Angiotensin-converting enzyme inhibitors (ACE inhibitors) such as: benazepril (Lotensin), enalapril (Vasotec), lisino-pril (Zestril), ramipril (Altace)

• Angiotensin receptor blockers (ARBs) such as: irbesartan (Avapro), losartan (Cozaar/Hyzaar), valsartan (Diovan)

Drugs to Lower Blood-Clotting Risk

• Aspirin

• Clopidogrel (Plavix)

For instance, taking an aspirin a day will lower risk of a heart attack or stroke by about 30 percent. We don't know which dose of aspirin is the best, so we tend to start with a low dose (or baby dose) of aspirin, which is usually 81 milligrams per day. (Be aware there also are enteric-coated versions that are gentler on the stomach, and aspirin with calcium for women.) For some patients who are at high risk for having a heart attack, or who have recently had a heart problem, the dose is increased to 325 mg per day (which is one adult-strength tablet). The problem with aspirin is that its action makes you bleed and bruise more easily. It also can be tough on the stomach, making you more prone to ulcers and other gastric abnormalities. But these problems occur at a low rate and are far outweighed by aspirin's benefits. If a patient, often a slender woman, is having problems with excessive bruising on aspirin given every day, I will just have her take it three days a week (usually Monday, Wednesday, and Friday, or only on even or odd days of the month).

---

*It turned out that everybody, no matter how low or
high their baseline cholesterol levels, had a reduced
risk for heart attack when taking a statin.*

Drugs such as statins (Zocor, Mevacor, Lipitor, Pravachol, Lescol, and Crestor) can lower your bad cholesterol and your risk of having a heart attack by 25 to 30 percent. Many of us consider statins an important tool in lowering the risk for heart disease in all patients with the metabolic syndrome and/or diabetes. One study, called the Heart Protection Study (HPS), looked at the value of giving people at high risk for heart disease a statin drug, regardless of the level of cholesterol. It turned out that everybody, no matter how low or high their baseline cholesterol levels, had a reduced risk for heart attack when taking a statin. Therefore, most physicians these days should recommend that you start on a statin drug if you have the metabolic syndrome.

Statins work by lowering the production of cholesterol in the body. (We all make cholesterol from our liver, in addition to the cholesterol we eat.) They have been used in millions of people since they were first introduced in 1987. The major side effects tend to be minor and include such things as an upset stomach or diarrhea. However, they can cause muscle pain, which at times can be quite significant. Let your doctor know if you feel increased muscle pain. Sometimes you can tolerate one statin and not another, so switching among them may be helpful. Very rarely this increase in muscle pain can cause the actual destruction of muscle tissue. This is very serious. It is called rhabdomyolysis, and it can lead to death. Fortunately, this almost never happens unless the statin is mixed with another drug, such as another type of cholesterol-lowering medication (Lopid, for instance), or drugs used for immunosuppression following transplant. Statins, like many drugs, can affect the liver. Although the harm to the liver is usually not permanent, you should have your liver tests monitored within three months of first starting on a statin and then every six months thereafter.

Drugs that lower triglyceride levels, such as Lopid and Tricor, can also lower your risk of having a heart attack. Although statins are generally chosen first, these drugs can also be beneficial. They have fairly few side effects and do not usually cause the muscle pain seen with the statins. But they, too, can cause problems in the liver and should be monitored just like the statins. If one of these must be combined with a statin, Tricor is preferable to Lopid, because Tricor seems less likely to cause any serious muscle breakdown.

We think that the ACE inhibitors reverse a low-level inflammation of the lining of your blood vessels—the kind of inflammation that increases the risk for developing cholesterol clogs and having heart attacks.

Two other types of drugs are considered vital to the treatment of the metabolic syndrome. These drugs initially were designed to lower blood pressure, but have turned out to have many other benefits as well. One class of these drugs is called angiotensin-converting enzyme (ACE) inhibitors. These ACE inhibitors work to inhibit the effect of an enzyme that converts angiotensin (a sort of hypertension hormone) into its active form, renin. The result is lower blood pressure, with the side benefit that the blood vessels throughout the body seem to become less irritated and inflamed.

These ACE inhibitors help the lining of the blood vessels become smoother. I tell patients that the lining of their blood vessels changes from being like sandpaper to Teflon and allows blood to flow more smoothly. We think that the ACE inhibitors reverse a low-level inflammation of the lining of your blood vessels—the kind of inflammation that increases the risk for developing cholesterol clogs and having heart attacks. The ACE inhibitors also seem to have the additional effect of helping the kidneys stay healthy.

Still, like all drugs, ACE inhibitors have side effects. The most common side effect is an annoying, dry cough. Although this is supposed to be uncommon, I see it often, especially in women. If someone develops a cough on an ACE inhibitor I switch them to an angiotensin receptor blocker (see below), which doesn't cause a cough. Sometimes when I switch people to a different drug, they think the new drug is causing the cough when it really isn't. It is the ACE inhibitor cough slowly going away, which can take up to a month. The other main side effect, which your doctor will look for with a blood test, is that these drugs can cause the potassium level in your blood to go up. If the potassium level goes up too high it can be dangerous, so you will need to have a blood test for this four to six weeks after starting on the drug.

The final group of drugs used in the treatment of metabolic syndrome is the angiotensin receptor blockers (ARBs). These drugs act a lot like ACE inhibitors, but they do their job differently. ARBs work by directly blocking the effects of renin on blood vessels, instead of blocking its production. Although we have less information on ARBs than ACE inhibitors (they haven't been around quite as long), they seem to have similar benefits. And in some cases, if someone is developing kidney failure, ACE inhibitors and ARBs can be combined together for added benefit. ARBs generally do not cause a cough, but they can cause an increase in potassium levels. You need to have these levels followed.

Interestingly, there are some studies in which statins and ACE inhibitors helped lower the rates for developing diabetes. Although this effect is not nearly as strong as with lifestyle change and physical activity, or with the glitazones, it still may be real.

Three Drugs You Should Take to Maximally Lower Your Risk for Heart Attack and Stroke

- Aspirin (81 mg per day or more)

- Statin

- ACE inhibitor or ARB

Medications Help Manage the Risk of Prediabetes

Medications can be extremely helpful in the management of prediabetes. Some drugs, like metformin and the glitazones (Actos and Avandia) are really drugs for treating type 2 diabetes. More and more studies are coming out that show these drugs may be useful for preventing diabetes as well. Obviously, it is important to use these medications along with the lifestyle changes (healthier diet, more physical activity) that are recommended for treating insulin resistance. Other drugs, such as statins, aspirin, ACE inhibitors, and ARBs, are designed to lower the risk for heart disease. Because prediabetes is a state of a higher-than-normal risk for heart disease, many people can benefit from taking these risk-lowering medications. Not long ago we didn't know how high the risk for heart disease was in people at risk for diabetes and, worse, we didn't know how to prevent it. In a few short years, I've gone from speaking mostly about the need to treat high blood sugar levels to urging prevention of the underlying problems in the first place.

I'm happy to be addressing prevention earlier and earlier because it allows me to make the greatest difference in people's lives. If you're at risk or have prediabetes, you can deal with diabetes prevention, too. You will never regret it.

PART THREE

UNDERSTANDING AND TREATING TYPE 2 DIABETES

NINE

TYPE 2 DIABETES: THE STEALTH DISEASE

Diabetes is the last thing on your mind when you go in for a routine physical or to talk with your gynecologist about entering menopause. You don't have any unusual symptoms, although you may be feeling a bit more tired than usual. So you are taken completely off guard a few days later when your doctor informs you that your tests have come back and that your blood sugar is elevated.

At this point, health care professionals generally proceed in one of two ways. Neither is good. One is to tell you that your sugar is a bit too high, but not to worry about it yet. The other is to suddenly, shockingly, tell you that you have diabetes and give you a prescription for some diabetes medication. Then you're told to come back in a month—all without any discussion of what diabetes is, the changes it will bring to your life, and what to expect in the future. If you currently have diabetes, is this how you found out?

There are other approaches, of course, depending on the doctor. Some do just the right thing by making sure you are appropriately diagnosed and informed about the disease and how to deal with it. But in busy doctors' offices this happens less often than it should.

If I were going to write a "bill of rights" for newly diagnosed diabetes patients, it would include just two simple, but crucial articles:

1. Any increase in blood sugar readings will be closely monitored, and the ramifications of the elevated levels explained until they are understood.

2. Any diagnosis of prediabetes or diabetes will be followed by:

a. Nutrition education (ideally with a nutritionist knowledgeable in diabetes)

b. Diabetes education (received either in a class or in individual sessions, or through reading books such as this one)

c. Close personal follow-up until you are comfortable with the elements of treatment and on the way to reaching targets for blood sugar, lipids, and blood pressure—however long that takes.

You don't have to give up bread and pasta for the rest of your life.

Being diagnosed with diabetes is almost always an emotional experience. You may have seen a family member suffer with diabetes or read how horrible diabetes can be. You may think that your life is over, at least life as you have known it. You are afraid that your familiar, comfortable habits will have to change. You feel guilty. You have been fighting your weight all of your life and now it causes you to have this horrible disease. The prospects for the future can be daunting and, sometimes, beyond overwhelming.

Often the response to this fear is denial, to pretend that your diabetes doesn't exist and that you can go on with your life as if nothing has happened. But that approach can kill you, or even worse, it can cause terrible problems before it kills you. What you may not know, may not have been told, is that nothing bad needs to happen to you if you can modify your eating and exercise habits a little. You don't have to give up bread and pasta for the rest of your life. You don't have to start working out like a professional athlete. What you do need to do is learn what behaviors really make the difference in living well with diabetes and how to incorporate them into your life. Give yourself permission to be human. One imperfect day or week of diabetes management won't cause you permanent harm. But one imperfect year just might.

Some newly diagnosed patients ask very few questions. This

makes treating them more difficult, as I never know what they are thinking or feeling. Others come armed with lists of concerns. Patients often bring a family member or friend with them to their initial appointment. I highly recommend this. When studies have been done to find out how much we learn in a doctor's appointment, it turns out that less than half of what is said sinks in. This would be especially true of someone still in shock from a diabetes diagnosis. Having a second pair of ears with you can double how much you remember afterward. In addition, I suggest you take notes. Written reminders of what was said and recommended will help you when you are at home, trying to figure out what you are supposed to do. An occasional patient will bring a tape recorder, which I don't mind. But in today's litigious world some physicians might feel uncomfortable and intimidated by this. Since your physician needs to be your ally, you want to be sure that any office visit is as relaxed and open as possible for both of you.

PREPARING YOURSELF FOR CHANGE

Before you learn how to take care of your newly diagnosed diabetes, it's important that you understand that you needn't be afraid. We all like our old habits; they're comfortable and familiar. And, yes, diabetes can radically affect your life: your spontaneity; how you spend your leisure time; how, what, when, and where you eat. Suddenly, instead of relaxing after a hard day's work, you are supposed to exercise. You have to prick your finger to test your blood sugar levels a number of times each day. You have to go to appointments with doctors, a nutritionist, and a diabetes educator, and take multiple pills every morning and evening. How can I tell you this is anything less than intrusive?

But try the following four concepts on for size. First, you should know that you probably have had a mild form of diabetes for five to seven years before you were officially diagnosed. That's how long we think most people with type 2 diabetes go before someone finally makes the diagnosis. This is neither your fault nor your doctor's, as doctors don't often know how to diagnose early diabetes. Even if they do, they often don't know what to do about it. Now that you know you have diabetes, I suggest you look ahead to the treatment taking effect. You're going to have more energy and will feel stronger than you have in a long while.

***Now that you know what you have,
you can do something about it.***

Second, you probably had an inkling way in the back of your mind that you were at risk for getting diabetes. Maybe someone in your family had diabetes, or you've been hearing about diabetes on the news and some of the symptoms mentioned sounded all too familiar. Regardless, now that you know what you have, *you can do something about it.* Instead of worrying in a general sense, you now have the power to confront and control your condition. There are many, many things you can do that will improve your quality of life, at least as far as diabetes goes.

Third, the changes you need to make will be incorporated slowly. You only have to lose a little weight each month, eat a little less carbohydrate with each meal, start exercising a little each day. It's a gradual hill to climb, not a mountain.

Fourth, you hopefully will never know the disaster of complications because if you're reading this book you already are taking control. The patients I see with complications have them mostly because they didn't have good diabetes care available to them. But sometimes it's because they weren't able to accept the changes they needed to make. You don't have to be one of these people. You can take care of your diabetes *now* and protect yourself from harm.

Don't think you can learn about diabetes all at once. You learn about it in increments, sometimes going back to a prior lesson before proceeding to the next one. And although I love it when patients are curious, I try to help them prioritize their questions. Some need to be answered right away, others should be saved until later. I tell patients that getting diabetes is a little like going to school. You don't expect to learn everything on the first day. You attend classes, read, and gradually master the material. Don't pressure yourself. Just learn what you need to know as you need to know it.

Adjusting to life with diabetes is a process. You should plan on seeing your physician several times, especially in the beginning, and visiting with a nutritionist, an educator, and going to classes. It takes a commitment right up front. But I can assure you if you put in the time in the beginning it pays off down the road. I know—you are probably busy. And of course you didn't plan on getting diabetes. No one does. But education early in the process can eliminate fears, not to mention complications, in the future. The learning part doesn't last forever; after a few weeks it is likely that you will know what you need to know and will be able to start coming in once every month or two instead of every week.

You won't feel much different if your blood sugar was 200 mg/dl instead of the normal 100.

WHAT IS TYPE 2 DIABETES?

Most people who get type 2 diabetes don't know what it is. Type 2 diabetes is both a genetic disease, one that almost always runs in families, and a disease of lifestyle, often (but not always) related to weight gain and inactivity. People with type 2 diabetes are always resistant to insulin. This means that insulin doesn't work as well as it should. Insulin is a hormone that transfers sugar into our cells. It also influences the breakdown of fat in our fat cells and regulates how much sugar and fat we have floating around our bloodstream. Insulin is the body's regulator of fuel. Too much insulin and our blood sugar level goes too low (and ultimately we could pass out from lack of sugar to our brain); too little insulin and our blood sugar levels go too high. Interestingly, our bodies don't really care, in the short term, if our blood sugar levels are too high. You won't feel much different if your blood sugar was 200 mg/dl instead of the normal 100. But while you may not feel that there is anything wrong, high blood sugar levels are damaging your eyes, your kidneys, your heart, and your nerves. This is why diabetes is called the "silent killer"—you can walk around with high blood sugar levels for years without knowing it.

When your body is resistant to insulin it means that it takes larger amounts of insulin to keep your sugar levels in the normal range

(100 mg/dl). The beta cells in your pancreas (the organ that makes insulin) keep making extra insulin in order to correct for the insulin resistance. (See figure in prediabetes chapter.) No one knows exactly what causes insulin resistance. There are lots of theories but no complete answers. Suffice it to say that we know it exists and can measure it by measuring increased insulin production in your body.

Getting older, gaining weight, being less active, having certain genetic predispositions, taking certain medications (such as prednisone), developing gestational diabetes during pregnancy, and illness increase insulin resistance. Conversely, losing weight, increasing exercise, and avoiding medications that worsen insulin resistance can improve insulin sensitivity.

In type 2 diabetes, the insulin resistance and increased demand on the beta cells cause the beta cells to burn out. In some people this insulin production failure happens sooner than in others. There are some people who are extremely overweight but who are fortunate enough not to have diabetes genes. These people are able to continue to make extra insulin forever. If you could look under a microscope at the beta cells of a person without diabetes, you'd see little bubbles of insulin waiting to be released. The beta cells of someone with diabetes look like they're covered with pink chewing gum. Not all of the beta cells are destroyed by this "gunk"— there are enough left to make some insulin, but only about half of what is needed.

Type 2 Diabetes = Insulin Resistance (cells don't respond normally to insulin) + Insulin Deficiency (not enough insulin)

DIAGNOSING TYPE 2 DIABETES

Blood Glucose Levels

Type 2 diabetes is diagnosed primarily by measuring an increase in the blood sugar levels in your body. We could measure insulin resistance or the production of insulin, but that is more involved and usually is not necessary. Sugar levels rise and fall; they are lowest before eating and rise after eating, particularly if you eat carbohydrate in the form of sugar or starch. Diabetes is diagnosed by measuring your blood sugar levels while you are fasting, which means you haven't eaten or drunk anything containing calories overnight (for ten to twelve hours). If your fasting blood sugar level is greater than 125 mg/dl, you have diabetes. A normal fasting blood sugar level for a person without diabetes is less than 100 mg/dl. It doesn't sound like that much of a difference, but it is significant.

This fasting blood test is supposed to be done twice, to confirm the diabetes diagnosis. Most of the time, though, it is done only once, especially if the level is very high and the diagnosis is obvious. If your doctor measures a *nonfasting* blood sugar level and it is more than 200 mg/dl, you also are very likely to have diabetes. People without diabetes never have blood sugar levels that are greater than 140 mg/dl, even after eating a sugary or high-starch carbohydrate. What you should remember as a simple frame of reference is the number 100. Your blood sugar levels should be less than that.

Sometimes your doctor will ask you to do an oral glucose tolerance test. You'll have your blood sugar level measured before drinking a super-sweet soda (usually either orange- or cola-flavored). Your blood sugar will then be measured again two hours later. Usually this test is not needed, except in pregnancy or if your doctor is trying to find out if you have early glucose intolerance (often measured in research studies). Glucose tolerance testing is necessarily inaccurate. It's just that the results you get on one day can vary widely from results on another. I myself rarely do this test on patients because I can generally learn what I need to know from other, less complicated and more reliable tests.

People without diabetes never have blood sugar levels that are greater than 140 mg/dl, even after eating a sugary or high-starch carbohydrate.

A1C Levels

Another test that is very helpful in the diagnosis of diabetes is the hemoglobin A1C (or simply, A1C). This is a test that measures your average blood sugar levels over time and it can be done at any time of day, fasting or not. Sugar sticks to your red blood cells and stays stuck for as long as the red blood cells live (which is about three months). The higher your blood sugar levels, the more sugar sticks. The A1C test correlates how much sugar is stuck to your red blood cells with average blood sugar level. This is a great way to tell what your blood sugar levels are day in and day out, since it reflects your blood sugar levels before and after eating for weeks at a time. A normal A1C level is 4 to 6 percent. If your A1C level is above normal at all you may have prediabetes or diabetes. And if your A1C is more than 7 percent diabetes is very likely.

The A1C test correlates how much sugar is stuck to your red blood cells with average blood sugar level.

For people with diabetes I recommend having their A1C level checked every three months. The closer the A1C level is to the normal range (4 to 6 percent) the lower the risk for having complications of diabetes. This is a number you can follow and that can change through treatment. Ask your doctor at every visit to tell you your A1C level; if it is above 7 percent, ask how you can lower it.

Fats and Cholesterol Levels in the Blood

Type 2 diabetes is commonly thought of only in relation to sugar levels, but it is a more complicated disease. Although people with type 2 diabetes do in fact have high blood sugar levels (which can cause all sorts of related problems), more people with diabetes actually die from heart disease. Having type 2 diabetes more than *doubles* your risk of heart attack. The main culprit is cholesterol. Increased risk for heart disease is present even if your blood cholesterol levels are fairly normal. While the reasons for this are unclear, we know that many people with type 2 diabetes have levels of

HDL (good) cholesterol that are too low and levels of triglycerides (fat in the blood) that are too high. We also think that diabetes causes the LDL (bad) cholesterol particles to be smaller and more dangerous. Therefore, it is very important to monitor your levels of cholesterol and triglycerides and treat them if they are abnormal. Also, be sure your doctor orders a fasting lipid panel, to measure total cholesterol, LDL, HDL, and triglyceride levels when you are first diagnosed with diabetes. You should be retested at least once a year after that.

---

*Having type 2 diabetes more than **doubles** your risk of heart attack.*

Kidney Function

Diabetes can affect your kidneys, the body's filtration system. At the time you are diagnosed with diabetes and every year after that you need to have at least two kidney function tests. The first one, the serum creatinine kidney test, involves taking a blood sample and measures how effectively your kidneys filter your blood. Ideally, this level is around 1.0 mg/dl, although usually anything below 1.4 in a female and 1.5 in a male is considered normal. Women tend to have lower creatinine levels than men do. Creatinine levels sometimes can go up if you are dehydrated (not drinking enough fluid). Once this level goes up, there is not much you can do to bring it down. It's essential to identify kidney damage early, when we can still make a difference.

The other kidney test, for prior damage, is a urine test to see if there is any leakage of protein from your kidneys into your urine. This leakage is the first sign of damage to your kidneys. If caught early, your doctor can prescribe medication to stop the condition from getting worse. It's an easy test—you simply need to pee into a cup in your doctor's office and then the sample is sent for testing. When kidney function is shown to be low, a further test requiring a twenty-four-hour collection of urine is indicated.

The kidney-related value in your urine that you want measured is called an albumin to creatinine ratio, or A/C ratio. Sometimes this is called a microalbumin test. What this tells you is how well your kidneys are working. The A/C ratio gives a sense of kidney effectiveness and degree of kidney damage. It's okay to lose a little albumin in your urine, but we also need to determine how much creatinine is being lost as well. We want to see much more creatinine in the urine in relation to protein that is being lost (if any). The result of this test should be a figure less than 30. If it is, your kidneys are working correctly.

The A/C ratio gives a sense of kidney effectiveness and degree of kidney damage.

Below is a list of common diabetes-related tests that *aren't* as helpful or as conclusive as the ones I recommend. Yes, these sound complicated, and indeed understanding diabetes *is* difficult, even for some doctors. But the point is, you need to know about this, and care about this, to understand the related physical elements of diabetic health. Catching kidney damage early is crucial.

1. *Urine protein test.* A special test stick is dipped into your urine and various patches on the stick turn a different color depending on the contents of your urine. If on this "dipstick test" you are positive, that *may* mean serious kidney damage. But it is more likely that you will be negative on a dipstick, particularly if you have just been diagnosed with diabetes. If a microalbumin test isn't done in conjunction with the dipstick test, you won't know whether or not you have any early kidney damage—the microalbumin test is always positive before the dipstick is.

2. *Creatinine clearance test.* This is a test done on a twenty-four-hour urine collection and tells you how well your kidneys function overall. But it *does not* tell you if any damage revealed is due to diabetes or some other cause.

3. *Other ratios or a measurement of "microalbumin" without a ratio.* Just be persistent in asking for an "albumin to creatinine

ratio" and once you get the number, check to be sure it is less than 30. If it is over 30, you are supposed to have the test repeated to confirm the results.

Blood Pressure

Blood pressure is a very important marker for those diagnosed with diabetes. Many studies have found that controlling blood pressure may be every bit as important, if not more important, than controlling blood sugar levels because of the potential for artery damage associated with diabetes. When your blood pressure is measured, be sure that the cuff used fits your arm. If you are a larger person, then a larger size cuff should be used. If you are smaller, then you may need a child-sized cuff. When you are having your blood pressure measured, be sure to sit still, with your legs uncrossed and arm held out naturally at the level of your heart.

Blood pressure for those with diabetes should be less than 130/80 mmHg. You can test your blood pressure at home—many of the home blood pressure machines are quite accurate. Blood pressure often is highest within ten minutes of waking up, but everyone has their own rises and falls throughout the day. One word of advice: Patients I see often say their blood pressure levels are higher in a doctor's office than they are at home (so-called white coat hypertension). I don't discount this assertion because many people find seeing doctors stressful. But if your blood pressure is high in a doctor's office, it is likely to be high at many other stressful times throughout the day. That type of high blood pressure can still lead to problems such as stroke, heart attack, and kidney damage. All of the studies on high blood pressure have used readings taken in medical centers; they weren't based on home readings. So nervous or not, a high blood pressure in a doctor's office may still portend problems if left untreated.

You can test your blood pressure at home—many of the home blood pressure machines are quite accurate.

PURSUING HEAD-TO-TOE HEALTH CARE

When you discover that you have diabetes, you need to find a number of health care providers to work with beyond a primary care physician and/or endocrinologist. In chapter 3 I discussed how to assemble a health care team, which should include at least two specialists—a podiatrist (foot doctor) and an ophthalmologist (eye doctor). Specialists, whom you may have to travel to see, play limited but essential roles in diabetes treatment. Like kickers in football or relief pitchers in baseball, they must be ready to come off the bench and into your game when they are needed. Preliminary exams of your feet and eyes, however, can be done by your primary physician.

Foot Exam

In diabetes you can develop what is called neuropathy, or loss of sensation in various areas of your body, particularly the feet. Before the nerves die and become numb, however, they often cause extreme pain. This pain is very hard to treat and is usually worse at night. By the time you can't feel your feet, your feet are abnormally vulnerable. For example, you can't tell if you have a cut or blister on your foot. This lack of pain is dangerous because pain is a warning sign of a problem. Therefore, if you lose sensation in your feet, you have to use your eyes instead of our nerves to detect problems. You need to examine your feet every morning and evening to be sure there are no cuts, sores, or infections that need to be looked after.

―――――

If you lose sensation in your feet, you have to use your eyes instead of your nerves to detect problems.

―――――

A foot exam from your health care provider should start with a general inspection of your feet. Your doctor should look at the tops and soles of your feet as well as between each of your toes for any cracks or sores. Then your pulses should be felt to make sure they are strong—one pulse point is on the top of your foot and another is on the inside, by your ankle. Next, your reflexes should be tested by tapping on your knees and ankles to see if you respond. Finally, you should have measurements done of how much sensation you have in your feet. The doctor may touch you with a light monofilament (sort of like stiff fishing line)—the best test of whether or not you can feel enough to protect your feet—or with a vibrating tuning fork. There are other tests that can be done, but in most cases, they aren't needed. What you do need to know is whether you have any signs of nerve damage and are at risk for developing problems in the future.

If your feet are found to be affected by diabetes, you may be referred to a podiatrist who can help give your feet special care. You should also have your health care provider point out anything that is not normal. When I tell patients to check their feet every day, most look blankly at me and ask, "What am I checking for?" So I try to show people what is normal and what I would worry about. Usually, it is a change, some sort of red spot or sore that is new and doesn't seem to be healing.

Eye Exam

High blood sugar levels can cause damage to the retina, which is the area inside the eye at the back. You actually can see the back of the eye by looking in through the front of the eye. The back of the eye is really the only place we can easily see blood vessels and nerves. High blood sugars can make tiny blood vessels in the retina break. The resulting leakage can damage the nerves and lead to blindness. But you can have serious damage to the back of your eye without any change in vision.

Any doctor can look at the back of your eye. But most of the time your pupil is too small to allow the doctor to see much. So you must go to an ophthalmologist (a doctor who specializes in diseases of the eye) to have a dilated eye exam. The eye doctor puts drops in your eyes to make the pupils enlarge, which allows a complete view of the retinal area. You should have a dilated eye exam every year. Sometimes the doctor will take pictures of the retina so that he or she can have something to check against at your next exam. Picking up changes early is very important because, as with all diabetic-related conditions, treatment is most helpful when damage is minor.

TABLE 9. TESTS AND TARGETS FOR TREATING DIABETES

Test	Treatment Goal
Fasting blood sugar level	80–130 mg/dl
A1C (overall blood sugar control)	Less than 7 percent
Lipid panel:	
Total cholesterol	Less than 200 mg/dl
LDL cholesterol	Less than 100 mg/dl (less than 70 mg/dl is ideal)
HDL cholesterol	More than 40 mg/dl
Triglycerides	Less than 150 mg/dl
Serum creatinine (kidney function)	Less than 1.4 mg/dl in females Less than 1.5 mg/dl in males
Urine albumin to creatinine (A/C) ratio (early test for kidney function)	Less than 30
Blood pressure	Less than 130/80 mmHg
Foot exam	To monitor any loss of sensation and treat any sores or cuts
Dilated eye exam	To treat any retinal damage

....

"In a strange way, I feel that getting diabetes was beneficial."

Howard's story of being diagnosed with diabetes is a classic one, with a few twists. Because he knows lots of doctors, he was able to ask good questions early and find answers that sent him to my office. But it was his own curiosity, determination, and persistence that have made the difference in his well-being.

One day I was playing golf with an orthopedic surgeon I know and I got a cramp in my hand from holding the club too tightly. He told me to drink a lot of orange juice, because I needed more potassium. So I started drinking orange juice. The more I drank, the more thirsty I became. And at night I couldn't go to sleep without having a glass of

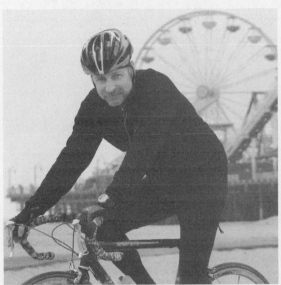

water by my bed. I also had to urinate all the time, day and night. And all of a sudden, overnight, my vision became so bad that I could barely see anything in front of me. I needed the highest power reading glasses I could buy at the store just to get around. I felt like I was under murky water.

Numerous people were telling me that I looked like I had lost weight. I thought they were all out of their minds because I had been at the same weight for many years. So I went out and bought a scale, which confirmed the fact that I was losing weight. However, I still didn't believe it, and bought another scale because I thought the first scale was wrong. Well, the scales were right. I was sick and didn't know it.

Of course, when this stuff starts happening to you, you are most aware of it when your doctors are not around—in the evening, or in the middle of the night when it's difficult to alleviate your fears. One evening, I couldn't take it anymore. I called my brother, the ophthalmologist, and explained what had been happening to me. He told me to find an all-night drugstore and go get a urine stick and test myself for glucose. I did, and the test was strongly positive for sugar. It was the result I most didn't want to see—even though my vision had gotten to the point where I needed my wife to see it for me. The next day many of my doctor friends came over to visit. They all had the same look and the same headshake when speaking to me about my symptoms.

I did an experiment and found out if you put sugar in a little bit of water, all of a sudden you have a thick syrupy substance. Then I started to understand that the more sugar that goes in, the stickier and the thicker that substance gets. I realized that every small vessel in my body was getting clogged. Then I started to understand why my parents both had open-heart surgery. All this contributed to my fear. The fear wasn't so much for myself, but more about how my family would be affected.

To conquer the fear I began asking questions. How did I get so out of control? When did this all actually start? I found my old medical records and saw that my fasting blood sugar levels had been running from 135 to 140 mg/dl for many years. Clearly, I had had diabetes and it was missed—or ignored.

I decided I needed a new doctor, so I called my brother again. He referred me to a recognized diabetes researcher. This researcher gave me the names of two physicians whom he had worked with and believed to be the best around. I spoke with the first one and my impression was of a businessman, more interested in himself than his patients. And then I got Dr. Peters.

What I like about Dr. Peters is that she seems to care less about money and more about her patients. She is always available to answer questions via e-mail or phone. In office visits, she spends all the time necessary with her patients. She motivated me to learn about diabetes.

I started to test my blood sugar levels and try to understand how everything I eat affects me. I found that carbohydrates affect me as much as sugar does. I met with a dietitian and started to really study what should be done. I learned that I needed to exercise and change my eating habits. It was very complicated for me, studying every piece of food and its contents. But this knowledge helped me understand my own reactions to food and exercise. So it was useful.

To eat right I had to figure out how to simplify the process for myself. One of the tricks that I used was to barbecue a lot of salmon, enough for my breakfasts for a couple of days. I enjoyed eating it, so I would get up in the morning, take a piece of the barbecued salmon, reheat it in the microwave, and have it with an apple or a pear and that would be my breakfast. I felt very satisfied with it and also I didn't have to worry about eating different things. For the rest of my meals, I tried to eat as much green stuff as I could and keep my carbs to a minimum. I ate fruit twice a day. I walked around with a bag of almonds and/or walnuts—salt free, I might add. There were days I felt like I was eating all the time.

The key to exercising was to find something I enjoyed doing and then do it every day. Bicycling was my choice. The hardest part was getting out of the door, so I had to make it fun for myself. I liked cycling, so it was a good carrot. I never really pushed myself in the beginning and I was so out of shape that it was embarrassing to see how little I was able to do. However, just the consistency of doing it every day made a difference. Before I knew it, I had a need and thirst to ride longer and longer and longer. Some days I would do more, some days I would do less—the main thing was to just get out there and do it. Finally, I was strong enough to ride one hundred miles at one time, from Los Angeles to San Diego. Other than having my family, this was the greatest achievement of my life.

My diabetes team helped me get through the minor barriers of misunderstanding that could have proven to be a total derailment. Sometimes these little details confuse you enough to totally set you off your goals and schedules. My doctor was there for me every step of the way. I always felt that no matter how basic a question was, the question would be treated with importance and answered with compassion and knowledge. I used my fear and the support I had to push me over the hurdles. In a strange way, I feel that getting diabetes was beneficial. It made me change my lifestyle and, maybe in my case, will even extend my life. The truth is, adapting to life with diabetes wasn't as hard as I thought it would be. It may sound weird, but I enjoyed the process. And for now the changes have made me the happiest I have ever been.

....

If you have been told your blood sugar level is high, first, don't panic. Second, don't ignore it. Go out and find the best medical care possible for you and for the sake of the people you love. You need to take charge of your health care and determine whether or not you have prediabetes or diabetes. In addition to having your sugar levels measured, you need to have your blood pressure checked, your blood fats (lipids) measured, and your kidney function assessed. If you are overweight and don't exercise much, it's a good opportunity to work with your health care team to get into shape. Medications may also be needed to lower your risk of developing the complications of diabetes.

It is within your power to prevent most of the diabetic complications, particularly if you continue to pay attention to your health and whether or not you are meeting and maintaining normal sugar, cholesterol, and blood pressure levels. You should do what Howard did: search for approaches to nutrition and exercise that resonate with your own way of living your life. A diagnosis of diabetes is a chance (unwanted as it may be) to face your health issues and improve how you feel.

TEN

GET REAL ABOUT NUTRITION AND EXERCISE

The greatest misconceptions about diabetes tend to revolve around nutrition. Partly this is because the advice doctors have given patients has changed over the years. And there's no shortage of wrong nutritional information being disseminated in popular culture. Most patients have already tried many different diets by the time they come to see me and most are frustrated because any success was short-lived. My intent is not to put you on yet another "diet." There is no diabetic diet. Rather, I want to show you how to develop healthier habits that you can follow for the rest of your life. In this book you can read more about nutrition in chapters 7 and 17, which will add to the information in this chapter. Each of those chapters looks at nutrition from a different diabetic perspective, although there is some intentional overlap to emphasize the key points.

There is no diabetic diet.

The single most important recommendation I can make to anyone with diabetes is to find a good nutritionist. You may think that you know a lot about nutrition because you've been on diets before, but what you need to know about living well with your particular type of diabetes is different. For one thing, the medications you are (or will be) taking will affect the nutritional advice that is right for you. You need an individualized meal plan—one that takes into account your own food preferences, goals, and health considerations. Even the American Diabetes Association has come to realize this. In the years since I have been working in the field of diabetes I have seen the ADA pendulum swing from having specific "diabetic diets" to recommending medical nutrition therapy based on individual needs. And that means working with a nutritionist.

Believe it or not, most doctors have had little or no training in nutrition. I went to one of the best medical schools in the country but I had no formal training in nutrition. I learned a lot about how the body works and doesn't work and how to treat diseases with medications, but almost nothing about the role of nutrition in health and illness. Many physicians think it is pointless to talk to patients about nutrition, because they're convinced the patients are never going to follow their advice anyway. But one thing I've learned as a physician (and as a mother) is that consistent, clear, and even repetitive advice often does help. Not everyone quits smoking the first time I bring it up, but stressing the importance of something such as stopping smoking or starting to exercise or losing weight can gradually sink in over time until it sticks. I think some of my patients must find my persistence annoying, but my consistent harping does make them exchange bad habits for good ones. And I always smile while I'm bugging them to, say, make an appointment with Meg, my nutritionist.

Many physicians think it is pointless to talk to patients about nutrition, because they're convinced the patients are never going to follow their advice anyway.

A good nutritionist can be very hard to find. Nutritionists who trained fifteen years ago or more may not know the newer approaches to diet therapy in diabetes. Younger nutritionists may not have a lot of experience that can tell them what does and doesn't work for a specific type of patient. When I was looking to hire a nutritionist for my diabetes center, I looked at more than fifty candidates before I found Meg Moreta. And although Meg has no magic formula in regard to weight loss, she has the elements that make a nutritionist excel: she has patience, is incredibly knowledgeable, and listens well. Meg is great at recommending small, specific manageable changes in diet and lifestyle, and if she doesn't know something she'll spend hours researching the answer. Perhaps her most important quality is that she is nonjudgmental. Patients love returning to her because she helps them feel good about the attempts they have made to change, small or large. She realizes diet modification is a gradual process, often without immediate results. The other thing she does, which I mentioned in chapter 7, is to assess each person's readiness to change. This allows her to teach at the right level. In other words, someone who is only *thinking* about changing needs different advice from someone who is already *making* substantial changes in their approach to food.

To understand nutrition you need to know that there are three basic classifications of foods we eat. They are: carbohydrates, protein, and fat. Carbohydrates are divided into two groups, the starchy carbohydrates (called "high-glycemic-index" or "high" carbohydrates) and the unlimited carbohydrates (called "low-glycemic-index" or "low" carbohydrates). The table below briefly describes the "big three." But read or review chapter 7 for more details.

Carbohydrates (high)	Potatoes, pasta, rice, grains, bread, fruit, milk, yogurt
Carbohydrates (low)	All vegetables (except corn, peas, beans, and potatoes, which are high carbs)
Protein	Meat, fish, eggs, chicken, cheese, soy
Fat	Oil, nuts, seeds, butter, margarine, salad dressing, avocados

SHOULD DR. ATKINS JOIN THE WEIGHT WATCHERS IN THE SOUTH BEACH ZONE?

The heading above is kind of a joke. But it does illustrate the confusion many people feel about the best way to lose weight. There are many, many commercial diets available. Are any of them applicable to type 2 diabetes?

If you are overweight, losing weight by any means will help treat your diabetes. Weight loss decreases insulin resistance and allows what insulin you are making to work more effectively, possibly bringing your blood sugar levels to normal. I have patients who've been diagnosed with diabetes who've lost 50 pounds and seen their high blood sugar levels fall to normal. If they keep the weight off, the diabetes stays away. However, they are always at risk (genetically) for developing it again. But no matter the dieting approach, it is amazing how useful losing weight can be for treating type 2 diabetes.

If you are overweight, there is really no one specific weight loss plan that works better than another.

While most people with type 2 diabetes are overweight, there is a smaller group of lean type 2s. We know less about lean people with type 2 diabetes, although we do know they have the same insulin resistance and insulin deficiency of overweight type 2 diabetics. In my experience, most of these thinner individuals will require both medication and a decrease in carbohydrate content to treat their diabetes. I will talk about the system of carbohydrate counting later, in chapter 17, but if you are lean and have type 2 diabetes remember that it is not losing weight that matters as much what you eat. So don't force yourself to become thinner than you should. Remember, each person with diabetes requires his or her own individual approach to eating, and lean people with diabetes are often the ones who most specifically need nutritional advice.

If you are overweight, there is really no one specific weight loss plan that works better than another. Scientific studies comparing most of the popular diets find that weight loss during the first six months is about the same. This means that you can lose weight following any weight reduction plan. The key is following it and changing your old eating habits.

I personally think that people with diabetes lose weight more easily when they eat less carbohydrate (starches, sugars—anything white). This doesn't mean eating no carbohydrate, as people do with the strict Atkins diet, but it means eating less, generally about 40 percent, of the diet as carbohydrate. This may be more in keeping with the popular South Beach diet. Choose more "natural" carbohydrates. Raw fruits and vegetables are better than fruits and vegetables that are cooked, mashed, pressed, pureed, baked, or altered in any way that affects their natural fibers and nutrients. The less processed the food, the better. So whole wheat bread is preferable to white bread, and brown rice is preferable to white rice.

Following the Atkins diet (or any high-protein, low-carbohydrate diet) probably doesn't hurt you in the short term and it makes it easier to lose weight. When you restrict carbohydrates and just burn fat and protein, your metabolism changes. You release ketones, the breakdown product of fat, into your bloodstream and these ketones help lower your feeling of hunger. When you aren't as hungry you eat less. And no matter the diet, it is eating fewer calories than you burn that leads to weight loss.

The less processed the food, the better.

The problem with the Atkins diet, or any diet that dramatically changes the way you eat, is that eventually you stop following it. That's simply human—none of us can stick to one rigid eating plan when the world beckons with a wide diversity of foods and flavors. But as soon as you start eating carbohydrates again, your hunger increases. So after a year on Atkins, most people have put their weight back on. This cycle of weight loss followed by weight gain is bad for your health, especially since many people often regain even more weight than they lost. My personal opinion about any high-protein diet is that you need to avoid eating too much saturated (bad) fat and cholesterol, which comes with eating more red meat. Your arteries have an immediate negative reaction if you load your bloodstream with too much unhealthy fat. Since having diabetes makes you extra vulnerable to having a heart attack or stroke I suggest keeping your arteries as healthy as possible.

———

This cycle of weight loss followed by weight gain is bad
for your health, especially since many people often regain
even more weight than they lost.

———

Why make the disruptive transition to an Atkins-type approach
and then another one later to a healthy maintenance diet? It
makes the most sense to take the one-step approach of changing
your eating habits permanently, in a way that you can fit into your
lifestyle. That way when you go out to eat or go to social events you
don't need to feel restricted and "different" from everyone else. If
you feel you need to jump-start your weight loss by following a
strict Atkins-type diet, no problem. But be prepared to shift to a
maintenance-style meal plan afterward. This means learning new
habits that are somewhere in between Atkins and your old habits.
Long-term success with weight reduction is really about changing
your *relationship* with food.

Other weight loss approaches work as well. Some people like to
be part of a group, such as Weight Watchers or Overeaters Anonymous. There are meal replacement programs where you buy special foods and you can even do some sort of partial liquid diet by
drinking Slim-Fast, Choice, or Glucerna for breakfast and lunch
and then eating a healthy dinner with protein, vegetables, and
salad. All of these methods help you lose weight, but won't necessarily help you keep it off permanently. That is where your nutritionist fits in. You need to learn how to balance your eating when
you are not on a strict diet plan, when you are back to living your
normal life.

Patients with type 2 diabetes who do best in the long term learn
how to eat less carbohydrate at each meal, and to eat meals with
a basic ratio of 40 percent carbohydrate, 30 percent healthy fat,
and 30 percent high-quality protein. Usually, these people eat five
times a day—each meal is smaller than normal and the two snacks
in between tend to be small, balanced snacks. This frequent eating helps keep hunger pains away, so you're not tempted to eat
doughnuts during your coffee break because you didn't eat breakfast and are starving by ten AM.

A long-term study called the National Weight Control Registry (NWCR) is currently being done by Drs. Rena Wing and James Hill. This is a study of people who were able to lose weight and keep it off. In the registry there are currently about three thousand patients, who have on average lost 60 pounds and kept it off for five years. About half of these people lost the weight on their own, without any type of formal program or help. Most of the people in the study had tried many times before to lose weight but kept gaining it back and more. Two-thirds had been overweight as children. What finally made them successful at losing weight and keeping it off was that something happened, a "hitting bottom," that prompted them to change. Sometimes this was seeing a loved one die from the complications of being overweight, or sometimes it was medical news about how much being overweight was hurting them. These patients made a decision to change their habits and then took action to make it happen.

What finally made them successful at losing weight and keeping it off was that something happened, a "hitting bottom," that prompted them to change.

Interestingly, the most common diet that most of them eat is a high-carbohydrate diet (not a high-protein diet, as I would have thought). Most eat small meals and snacks five times per day. Most eat breakfast every day. Almost all are physically active and they weigh themselves often to be sure they are not gaining the weight back. The most common form of physical activity is walking. They have also learned to eat in a way that keeps them from feeling deprived: they still eat the foods that are "bad" (the cakes, candy, and French fries)—they just eat less of them. This particular diet approach may not be right for everyone. I have met many people who must avoid eating any tempting foods at all, as they find that one small bite leads uncontrollably to a bigger portion. To find out more information about this registry, or to see if you can join, go to: www.uchsc.edu/nutrition/WyattJortberg/nwcr.htm and www.lifespan.org/Services/BMed/Wt_loss/NWCR/default.htm.

These success stories show us that a balanced approach works the best. Adherence to restrictive, deprivation diets ultimately doesn't last. Diet fads and food programs are very profitable, and obviously are filling an emotional need for a certain part of the American population. Common sense, balance, and moderation, while not as "sexy" as jumping on the newest diet bandwagon, may prove to be the way to go.

SUGAR IS NOT THE ENEMY

When people get diabetes they think that high sugar levels in their blood mean that they've been eating too much sugar. This is only partly true. Sugar in your bloodstream comes from two sources—carbohydrate and protein. Your body converts the carbohydrate in your diet into the sugar it needs to power your brain and body. If you don't eat enough of some form of sugar/carbohydrate, your body will make sugar by converting protein into sugar in your liver. Therefore, to simply stop eating sugar won't make your blood sugar levels normal. What you need to do is to find a balance between the carbohydrate, protein, and fat that you eat. This will help control your blood sugar levels and make weight loss possible (if you are overweight).

*All starches are carbohydrates,
but not all carbs are starches.*

The simple sugar we eat (for example, candy) is just another form of carbohydrate to our bodies. Carbohydrates include everything from table sugar to fruit, pasta to potatoes. Certain carbs are more intense and are grouped as starches. Rice, potatoes, and pasta belong in this category. All starches are carbohydrates, but not all carbs are starches. Starches are long chains of sugar molecules; table sugar is shorter chains. Whether a carb or a starch, all are broken down in our intestines as they are absorbed and all enter our bloodstream as sugar. Some sugar is absorbed more quickly—such as the sugar in soda and juice. Other sugar is absorbed more slowly, for example, the sugar in raw fruits and vegetables. How quickly a sugar is absorbed depends on the form the sugar is in; processed foods lead to a more rapid increase in sugar levels and raw foods to a lower rate of absorption. High-fiber foods, for example, lead to sugar that is more slowly absorbed.

The speed with which the sugar in food is absorbed by the body is described by the food's "glycemic index." A low glycemic index (defined as less than 55) means that the sugar is absorbed more slowly. A high glycemic index (more than 70) indicates a more rapidly absorbed food. When monitoring your carbohydrate intake, which really is the same thing as counting how much sugar you're consuming, it helps to know not only the total amount of sugar, but also the glycemic index of the foods you eat (visit http://www.diabetes.ca/Section_About/glycemic.asp). People with diabetes develop an intuitive "food sense" over time and learn how certain foods affect their blood sugar.

How quickly a sugar is absorbed depends on the form the sugar is in; processed foods lead to a more rapid increase in sugar levels and raw foods to a lower rate of absorption.

The truth is, you don't really need to know the glycemic index of brown rice versus white rice, although it is helpful to know that brown rice is better for you. A nutritionist can help you wade through all the terminology and give you pointers and simple, easy-to-remember guidelines. There are also many books that give you the calorie and carbohydrate breakdown of foods. I like the The Doctor's Pocket Calorie, Fat, and Carbohydrate Counter (2004 edition), mostly because it is small and simple to use. You can also go to a related website at www.calorieking.com. The website has a carbohydrate calculator that you can use to help you learn about the amounts of carbohydrate in various foods.

People with diabetes develop an intuitive "food sense" over time and learn how certain foods affect their blood sugar.

TABLE 10. CARBOHYDRATE FACTS

Source	Portion Size	Carbohydrate (grams)	Glycemic Index <55: low 55–70: moderate >70: high
Baked potato	1 medium/4 oz	30 g	85
Mashed potato	½ cup/4 oz	20 g	70
Sweet potato	3 oz	20g	51
French fries	4 fries/3 oz	46 g	75
Pita bread	6.5 inch/2 oz	35 g	57
White rice	⅓ cup cooked	42 g	72
Brown rice	1 cup cooked	37 g	55
White bread	1 slice/1 oz	12 g	70
Corn tortilla	2 shells/1 oz	17 g	68
Spaghetti (white)	1 cup cooked/6 oz	52 g	41
Spaghetti (whole wheat)	1 cup cooked/6 oz	48 g	37
Oatmeal (old-fashioned)	½ cup cooked/4 oz	12 g	49
Pretzels	1 oz	22 g	83
Peanuts (roasted)	½ cup/2.5 oz	16 g	14
Orange	1 medium/4 oz	10 g	44
Apple	1 small/5 oz	18 g	38

Here is an example of how you can change your breakfast to include more fiber and lower the glycemic index:

Breakfast #1: High glycemic index, low fiber, quickly absorbed carbohydrate

Corn flakes (1 cup)	25 g carbs	1.0 g fiber
1% milk (½ cup)	6 g carbs	
Orange juice (¾ cup)	20 g carbs	0.4 g fiber
Tea		
Total	*51 g carbs*	*1.4 g fiber*

Breakfast #2: Lower glycemic index, higher fiber, more slowly absorbed carbohydrate

Oatmeal (¾ cup)	27 g carbs	4 g fiber
1% milk (½ cup)	6 g carbs	
Blueberries (¾ cup)	15 g carbs	3 g fiber
Tea		
Total	*48 g carbs*	*7 g fiber*

Making Sugar from Protein

The liver is the source of most of the sugar the body makes. For example, during the night your liver is making enough sugar to keep your blood sugar levels normal as you sleep. If it didn't, you would either have to be up all night eating or you would wake up with a very low blood sugar level. This regulation becomes disrupted in type 2 diabetes. The insulin resistance causes the liver to make excessive amounts of sugar overnight, causing you to awaken with a sugar level that is way too high.

The liver can increase blood sugar levels in several ways. After eating carbohydrates, the liver stores the resulting sugar in its cells. It breaks down this stored sugar and releases it into your bloodstream. These sugar stores generally last for a few hours, then your liver shifts to making sugar from protein. This is how it is possible to maintain a normal sugar level on a high-protein diet; protein replaces carbohydrate as the primary source of sugar. If you don't eat enough carbohydrate and protein, your body will turn to another source of protein to break down—your muscles. If this persisted, you would essentially be starving yourself, which obviously wouldn't be healthy. You want to lose fat, not your muscle mass.

WHAT ARE MY WEIGHT LOSS GOALS?

I work with my patients to help them set goals as they start to lose weight. The goals I suggest for you are the same as for them:

1. Find a way to eat differently, so that you lose weight and feel satisfied.

2. Learn to incorporate increased physical activity in a consistent way into your lifestyle.

3. Understand how food affects your blood sugar levels.

4. Know how you can use diet and exercise to control your diabetes.

5. Improve your overall health. You may feel more attractive as well, but remember, we're striving for health.

When it comes to weight loss, you know better than anyone what is possible. I usually don't look at height and weight charts. I ask people what their lowest and highest adult weights have been and then I help them set a weight goal. I try to set achievable targets. The real goal is to slowly, gradually, lose weight and not regain it. It may, for instance, be possible for someone now wearing a size 12 to eventually fit into a size 6. But if they are a lot bigger, then it may be less achievable, and therefore not a good goal to set. As I've previously mentioned, losing 15 to 20 pounds can lower your blood sugar levels significantly and make you much healthier. The blood sugar response I see can be quite variable, however. If you have had diabetes for a long time or your initial blood sugar levels are over 300, you may not see as rapid a fall in blood sugar levels. Some of the medications I'll talk about later make weight loss harder but they improve blood sugar levels. It always comes down to establishing a balance between losing weight and making sure blood sugar levels are normal. Just remember, dropping extra pounds will always help your diabetes if you are overweight, no matter what your blood sugar levels or what medication you are on.

When I see a patient who has just been diagnosed with diabetes I view it as an opportunity to make lifelong changes. So should you. That drastic health upheaval can be a powerful motivator for weight loss. Many of my colleagues just shake their heads and think "they won't lose weight." Often, that's true. But I think that it is *possible* for people to lose weight so I give them a chance. Once people start on oral medications they often feel defeated, or they decide not to bother modifying their lifestyles. Or, occasionally the diagnosis isn't new. Some patients I see have been treated by another physician for years. For them, changing doctors can be another opportunity for motivation. It lets people see themselves and their diabetes from a different and perhaps more hopeful perspective.

Marc's story below touches on some of the obstacles that must be overcome in trying to change old habits. But, as you'll read, he persuaded himself to adopt a healthy lifestyle, and shares some wonderful tips based on his experiences living with diabetes.

....

"Food was love. Food was happiness. Food was family. Food was a reward."

I am fifty-nine years old and was a cable TV entrepreneur for more than thirty years. While chairing the National Cable Television Convention in Chicago in June 1999, I became extremely thirsty and very tired. A week later, I was diagnosed with type 2 diabetes.

The diagnosis of diabetes came as a particular shock because I love food and was afraid I'd lose that pleasure. My mom was a great cook. She made lots of wonderful foods for me when I was growing up and I developed a passion for food. Roast beef, cheeseburgers, pizza, French fries, bread, pasta, hot dogs, fried chicken, and lots of sweets. Food was love. Food was happiness. Food was family. Food was a reward.

In spite of this rather indulgent diet, I stayed slim. When I got married at twenty-two, I was 6'1" and weighed 130 pounds. I never thought that I would gain weight. It never occurred to me that I could end up with diabetes, even though both of my grandfathers had it, as

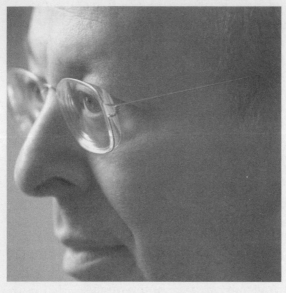

did members of my immediate family.

But I did gain weight. When I was first diagnosed with diabetes I weighed 220 pounds and did little exercise. My first reaction to the news was panic. I thought I could never eat the foods that I loved again. I would have to go on insulin and my health would rapidly deteriorate. I became mildly depressed. My wife, my kids, and my doctor tried to talk me out of the funk. Nothing worked until I decided to take control of my life and change my lifestyle to cope with my disease.

With the help of my doctor and a very knowledgeable nutritionist, Susan Dopart, we were able to devise a meal plan that worked for me. I still miss those French fries, but I adjusted my eating habits. It is not a diet, per se. It is the way that I must eat for the rest of my life. It is important to monitor what you eat and write everything down. If you cheat, you cheat yourself, not anyone else.

I am not a saint about my diet, but I have developed a few tricks to help. For instance, if I ever get a craving for something on a menu when I am eating out I tell myself that I have eaten that dish a thousand times in my life and I remember what it tastes like. Now, if I want a long life, I try something else.

Another bit of good advice is to read labels, but forget about calories. Look at protein grams (not percentages) and carbohydrates. Try to eat foods that are higher in protein grams than carbohydrate grams. The calories will take care of themselves when you watch what you eat. Weigh yourself at the beginning and end of the month. Become knowledgeable about food and the effect it has on your individual glucose levels.

When I first started working with my nutritionist, she taught me how to plan my meals. I learned the basic principles of how to eat correctly and then figured out how to use those rules whenever I ate, whether at home or when traveling. We broke down each meal into how much protein, carbohydrate, and fat I should eat. (Another tip: Watch the fat, particularly bad fats—those from animal fats or oils in processed foods—when you have diabetes.) Then I made lists of sample diets, with food that I liked, so I could understand what meals should look like. Here, for instance, is a list of snacks that I started to keep in the house in case of cravings:

- *String cheese*

- *Unsalted nuts (almonds, walnuts, peanuts)*

- *Soy nuts*

- *Crab and shrimp*

- *Sardines*

- *Tuna and salmon*

- *Hard-boiled eggs*

- *Canned chicken breast*

- *Cottage cheese*

- *Balance Bars or other low-carb food bars*

In addition to trying to increase my protein intake as well as my intake of vegetables and healthy carbohydrates, I also started to exercise. At first I started slowly, but was convinced by my physician and nutritionist that I needed to exercise six days a week in order to stay healthy. After a while it became a habit. I also found that I liked yoga, so I added it to my routine. Here is what my exercise routine looks like:

Monday, Wednesday, and Friday

- *30 minutes cardio in gym (treadmill, bike, rowing)*

- *30 minutes light weights and strength building (particularly legs)*

Tuesday and Thursday

- *40-minute morning walk before breakfast*

- *40-minute yoga session in the afternoon (power) or 40 minutes on the treadmill*

Saturday

- *1- to 2-hour bike ride or hike*

Sunday

- *Rest (sometimes I walk anyway)*

One of the hardest things I had to face was the need to check my blood sugar. I always hated having my blood taken. I used to avoid blood tests. I would break out in a cold sweat and once almost fainted on the doctor's table. You can imagine my delight when I was first diagnosed with diabetes. A blood phobic, having to prick his finger twice a day? No way!

Well, I did it. It turned out to be no big deal. For the first month, I just stared at the little vampire kit. I got one of those adjustable lancets (you set the needle level) and then I found a smaller lancing device, which made taking blood from my little finger easier. Finally, I just did it and I have been recording my blood ever since. I still do not like to give a blood sample at the doctor's office, but believe me, pricking your finger is okay and it doesn't hurt . . . much.

You need to do your own chronicling of yourself and of the disease. Therefore, you need a daily record of what you eat and how much exercise you do. If you want, you can keep track of your carbs and units, but I do not. I was fifty-four and weighed 220 pounds when I was diagnosed with diabetes. I have used my record book, along with some oral medication and my type A personality to lower my weight to 192, and to commit to exercise six days a week. My blood sugar levels are now so normal that my doctor says it's hard to find that I have diabetes. If I can do it, so can you. It may seem hard but, trust me, it is possible. And for the rest of your life you'll be proud that you learned to take charge of your diabetes.

....

EXERCISE AS A WAY OF LIFE

If you're like most people nowadays, you need to increase the amount of physical activity you do. This doesn't mean you have to become an aerobics fanatic. Marc, in the story above, had a hard time believing he could learn to exercise on a regular basis, but now he's grown used to it. Look at the benefits: Exercise will lower your blood sugar levels, decrease your risk of a heart attack, and lower your blood pressure. It is also a critical element in any weight loss plan.

So what's the problem, other than you "hate to exercise" or "don't have a spare minute" or are "just too tired"? I don't accept those excuses from my patients and always start them off with very small increments of exercise. For example, walk for five minutes, turn around, and walk back . . . you just completed a ten-minute walk! If you try to do too much too soon you will hurt yourself; the injury will be frustrating and will give you yet another reason not to exercise.

If you are over thirty-five you need to check with your primary physician to be sure it is okay for you to start exercising. You may want to (or have to) take a treadmill test. This test evaluates the blood flow in the arteries to your heart. If there is a problem, increasing exercise could cause a heart attack. It's important to pick up any abnormalities as early as possible, so you can get them treated *before* you have any real problems. I also recommend checking to make sure your eye exams are up to date because exercise can complicate untreated diabetic eye damage.

My goal—for you, for me, and for every adult—is to exercise for one hour a day at least five days a week. Do I reach this goal every week? Not always—I get too busy, or I feel sick, tired, and just bored with exercise. Sometimes I take a break. But overall, week in and week out, there are enough times that I do exercise to stay healthy. What is important to remember about exercise is that you can't let a bad day or a bad week or even a bad month send you completely off track. This applies to dieting as well. Both processes are marathons, not sprints. You just start up again, as soon as you can. I have made a commitment to myself and to my patients to exercise. If they have to do it to be healthy, so do I. Many people find an exercise buddy or join groups for the support. There are many options; experiment to find what is right for you in terms of a time, place, and way to exercise. Some people like to exercise at home; others prefer going to a gym. It may take some trial-and-error with different approaches to find the best one for you. But there is one that will work—perhaps many.

What is important to remember about exercise is that you can't let a bad day or a bad week or even a bad month send you completely off track.

Prepare to deal with obstacles, to counter your own internal arguments against exercising. Does it take too much time to go out for exercise? Buy a home machine, like a treadmill or exercise bike. Of course, that brings up another whole set of obstacles. I'll bet most Exercycles are used more often for hanging clothes than riding. (Sound familiar?) One issue you may face is that home exercise equipment is often not as good as the more expensive models found in gyms. Look at exercise equipment as a tool for health. Because it will be used over and over again, I recommend spending the money for a good machine. You can often find (barely) used ones in want ads or online. If you've never used exercise equipment before, it may be a good idea to join a gym or YMCA for a while to see which machines you like before buying one. Many gyms also have personal trainers available to instruct you on proper form and usage of the machines. Another issue that often comes up is lack of space at home for exercise equipment. My personal belief is that health should always come before interior décor. This certainly is true in my house.

Regardless of the type of exercise you choose, you should strive for forty-five minutes of aerobic activity (walking, swimming, cycling, running, rowing, etc.) and fifteen minutes of strength training (lifting light weights and stretching). If you haven't been exercising regularly you will need to work up to these time goals in small steps, maybe five to ten minutes a day for the first week, increasing in five-minute intervals as you become better conditioned. Try to stretch before you exercise, so you are less stiff warming up. As you increase exercise time, you also can increase the speed and intensity of exercise. If you walk for exercise you may want to buy a pedometer, so you can count your steps. The goal would be to take ten thousand steps per day to be healthy. Sound like a lot of walking? Well, remember the old saying: The longest journey begins with one step.

THE DYNAMIC DUO: EXERCISE *AND* DIET

You now know that exercise lowers insulin resistance and should reduce your blood sugar levels. When I look at people's blood sugar logbooks I often can see the effects of exercise in graphic fashion. Blood sugars are lower on exercise days and higher on days with less movement. I have patients who even use this exercise effect to "burn off" a carbohydrate-rich meal and bring an elevated blood sugar level back down. But don't forget that exercise and diet are complementary. In my experience with my patients, exercise without weight loss does not lower blood sugar levels enough to treat diabetes. Which is not to say that exercise doesn't help—it helps in all sorts of ways, particularly because it aids your heart and blood vessels. Also, sometimes there are mixed results in people who are very insulin resistant. But don't be discouraged if you start exercising and don't see an immediate fall in your blood sugar levels. Exercise *is* helping. Combining exercise with your nutrition plan is the best way to improve your overall health.

WEIGHT LOSS PILLS

Just as there is no magic diet plan, there is no magic weight loss pill. Fen-phen came the closest, but it caused such serious problems it was pulled off the market. It also had the downside of working only while you took the pills. Most people saw their weight loss reversed when they stopped the pills. We now have Meridia, which helps some people lose a little weight—around ten pounds. Meridia works to help you feel less hungry. The main side effects are that it can increase your blood pressure and it can also make you feel a bit spacey. My patients have reported limited success with it, but I'm always willing to let individuals who have good blood pressure try it. Like fen-phen, Meridia controls weight only as long as you take it;

the weight will come back once you stop using it. Meridia is expensive and not all insurance companies are willing to pay for it. For most people dropping ten pounds isn't unimaginable if they're watching their diet and exercising regularly—and the effects of losing the weight the old-fashioned way tend to be longer lasting. So you have to ask yourself, then: How much is ten pounds worth?

Another drug is the fat blocker Xenical. It stops the absorption of fat from your intestines. I almost never recommend Xenical because patients don't like the nasty side effect of leaky stool. On the other hand, it does work. It can cause some weight loss, and studies have shown that, like any weight loss treatment, it helps lower blood sugar levels.

I think there must be a million herbal preparations out there to help with weight loss. In my experience, none works particularly well, although if there is one food group that could be considered a "magic bullet," it would be fiber. When we conduct clinical trials we always use a placebo group. These participants get a sugar pill instead of medication, but they don't know that. The psychological effect of believing that you are taking some new drug that will help works in 20 percent of the group. A new drug needs to show an improvement over this placebo effect to be considered an improvement. Could this be what is happening with herbal supplements? It is hard to say. Mostly, I just want to be sure that there is nothing harmful about them. If they work—for whatever reason—in a given individual, great. Still, I always have my patients bring in all of their supplements so I can look at the bottles and check for safety. I don't have an herbal product to recommend, however, since I've never seen one with a consistent benefit.

OBESITY SURGERY

If you are very heavy (usually with a body mass index of more than 35) and have unsuccessfully tried a variety of different diets, obesity surgery may be an option for you. Although I personally know people who have had obesity surgery, almost none of my patients choose it. Obesity surgery generally works. It helps people lose weight and is very effective at lowering blood sugar levels. It surprises me that more of my patients don't consider the procedure.

It could be that they prefer not to risk the downside of complications after surgery, including infections, blood clots, and even death.

If you are considering surgical treatment for obesity, research it very carefully. Find the surgeon in your area who does the most procedures and talk with him or her about the different types of surgery available. Some operations are safer than others, while some are more effective at helping with weight loss. In addition to finding an experienced surgeon and reviewing the possible procedures, you need to ask about the recovery period and what to expect. Finally, you'll need to carefully review your insurance benefits. Some insurance plans will pay for the surgery, but only after very specific requirements have been met. The surgeon's office will often be experienced with these issues. But be sure to research it yourself, so you don't end up with a bigger than expected bill.

MONITORING YOUR PROGRESS

There are many ways to monitor the progress of a new nutrition and physical activity program. And there *will* be progress. But don't expect sudden miracles. You can't undo years of poor eating and inactivity overnight. Small changes over time will lead to improved health and new patterns that will stay with you for a lifetime. Gradually, over time, you will feel better and healthier. Your clothes will be looser, people will tell you that you look great, and you will have more energy.

Think about keeping a food log, which is a good way to know how much you are eating and when. These logs, which track what and how much you eat and when, are very helpful in communicating with your nutritionist. An example of such a log is shown below. What we want you to do is to record the details of what you consume. You also note when you exercise and for how long. Blood sugar levels are input from time to time so you can learn how your body responds to changes of food and exercise. You can keep track of your weight, but to avoid discouragement don't weigh yourself every day. Once a week seems reasonable for most people. It doesn't matter at this stage if weight loss is slow or nonexistent as long as you are exercising regularly and consciously trying to

BLOOD GLUCOSE AND LIFESTYLE DIARY

Date: ____

	3 AM	Fasting	Before Breakfast	After Breakfast	Before Lunch	After Lunch	Before Dinner	After Dinner	Bedtime
Time									
Blood glucose									
Insulin									

Exercise: Time: ____ **Duration:** ____ **Type (circle one):** Aerobic or weights
Stress:
Illness:

	Breakfast	Snack	Lunch	Snack	Dinner	Snack
Time						
Food eaten:						
Grams of CHO:						

adopt new habits. This is only a temporary system; you won't have to log everything for the rest of your life.

If you don't like the log shown here, you can use any log format you'd like (or design your own on your computer). The information just has to be clear and easily shared with your nutritionist.

TESTING BLOOD SUGAR LEVELS ON YOUR OWN

Testing your blood sugar levels is not always recommended when you are treating your diabetes with diet and exercise alone. I like it, though, and think that testing is a useful way to understand the effects of carbohydrates and exercise. There are many different meters available for testing your blood sugar levels. What they require is that you prick your finger with a lancet to obtain a drop of blood. (The lancet generally is inserted in a spring-loaded penlike device.) The blood is then put on a strip that goes into a glucose meter. Many of the meters read your blood sugar level quite quickly, often within six seconds, and require only a very small amount of blood. You will need to work with your diabetes educator to pick the meter that is right for you; this is sometimes dictated by what your insurance will allow. All meters come with instruction manuals and some come with instructional videos so you use the right technique. Most are very easy to use. Be sure that the vial your test strips come in is closed and dry. Strips have expiration dates and can go bad if exposed to the air. Also be sure that the code on your strip container matches the code shown on the meter (if this step is required). Finally, setting the date and time correctly makes it easier for us to understand the test numbers stored in your meter when you come in for appointments.

If your blood sugar level starts out well first thing in the morning, it is likely to stay reasonably well controlled throughout the rest of the day.

By testing your blood sugar levels first thing in the morning, you can tell how much sugar your liver is making overnight. This is called your "fasting" blood sugar level and should be 90 to 130 mg/dl. If your blood sugar level starts out well first thing in the morning, it is likely to stay reasonably well controlled throughout the rest of the day. Patients on diet therapy would do well to test their fasting blood sugar levels approximately three times per week to get an idea of how weight loss and exercise are affecting their diabetes overall. Testing blood sugar two hours after eating is useful as well. This can teach you how your body reacts to various foods. You can also test to compare a healthy meal with fewer carbohydrates and then after you've had pasta or rice, to see the difference in your blood sugar levels. You will learn the foods (or restaurant dishes) that cause your blood sugar levels to increase more than others, and can begin to fine-tune your own diet. I will often recommend the following pattern of testing to my patients: after breakfast on one day; after lunch the next day; after dinner the next; and so on. You can also test before and after exercise, or test after a meal and then again after exercise, to see how much each type of exercise lowers your blood sugar level. The more you test, the better your control.

Always leave some food on your plate.

NUTRITION BASICS FOR TYPE 2 DIABETES

The simple principles of diabetes nutrition are these: Eat small, frequent meals that include fat, protein, and carbohydrate in correct proportions. Avoid refined foods (sugar, white flour, white rice) and increase natural, less processed foods. Eat lots of fruits and vegetables, but don't drink your carbohydrates (that is, avoid fruit juices and soda). Read food labels carefully and be especially cautious of foods proclaiming they are low-fat—that may be true, but they more than likely are high in sugar or sodium content. Watch portion sizes, and in general eat 30 to 60 grams of carbs per meal (but not less than 100 grams of carbs per day, especially if you are physically active). Always leave some food on your plate. Wine in moderation is probably good for you; regular beer has too many carbs. Just say no to dessert. And, finally, burn more calories than you eat if you need to lose weight. You can go a long way toward accomplishing this by exercising forty-five to sixty minutes per day, five days a week (although you should start slowly and build up to that schedule). Exercise should be done by everyone, whether or not they need to lose weight. If you follow these rules you will feel better and your blood sugar levels will greatly improve. But they may improve even more when the proper medication is added to your regimen, as you'll learn about in the next chapter.

ELEVEN

USING PILLS TO TREAT DIABETES

There was a time I only had one type of oral medication to pre-scribe for treating type 2 diabetes. In the last couple of decades, however, the number of pills for diabetes treatment has increased steadily. I feel like a chef sometimes, mixing and matching the in-gredients of successful diabetes treatment. But the outcomes really are wonderful if the right mix is found.

HOW ORAL MEDICATIONS WORK

To understand how medications for type 2 diabetes work, you need to consider the two physiological components of type 2 dia-betes: insulin resistance plus insulin deficiency. Insulin resistance can be lowered through weight loss and exercise. Insulin defi-ciency can't be directly treated this way, but by reducing insulin re-sistance the body has to make less insulin to keep blood sugar levels normal. Lowering insulin resistance, then, puts less strain on your body to make insulin, and therefore insulin-making cells won't burn out as quickly. In other words, lowering insulin resis-tance lessens insulin deficiency. It's like trading in your SUV for a compact car. The compact uses gasoline more efficiently (lower the insulin resistance) and you need less gas (less insulin).

The treatment of first resort for type 2 diabetes always is diet and exercise because, as noted above, they are the two basic ways to lower insulin resistance. Before the current crop of oral medi-cations was available for treating insulin resistance the only alterna-tives were pills that increased insulin secretion, or insulin injections.

Then, starting in about 1996—relatively recently, really—several new types of medications were released (metformin and the glitazones). These medications worked to lower insulin resistance, creating more type 2 diabetes treatment options.

Below are listed the different basic treatment options, followed by discussion of their usage and how they can be combined for the best results. (Insulin shots are covered in the next chapter.) Once you understand your options, not only can you ask your doctor better questions, you can be a better participant in your own treatment.

To Increase Insulin Secretion

- Take a sulfonylurea agent (glyburide, glipizide, Glynase, Glucotrol, Micronase, Glucotrol XL, Amaryl)

- Take a meglitinide (Prandin or Starlix)

To Lower Insulin Resistance

- Lose weight

- Increase exercise

- Take metformin (Glucophage)

- Take a glitazone (Actos or Avandia)

To Limit Glucose Absorption

- Take an alpha-glucosidase inhibitor (Precose or Glyset)

To Increase Insulin Levels Directly

- Take insulin shots

To Increase Gut Hormones
(not yet available but the next new class of diabetes drug)

- Exenatide

- Liraglutide

- LAF 237 (DPP4 inhibitor)

TABLE 11. ORAL MEDICATIONS TO TREAT TYPE 2 DIABETES

Class	Generic Names	Trade Names	Can It Cause Low Blood Sugar Reactions?	Common Side Effects and Warnings
Sulfonylurea agents (SAs)	glyburide, glipizide, chlorpropamide, glimperimide	Micronase, DiaBeta, Glynase, Glucotrol, Glucotrol XL, Diabinese, Amaryl	Yes	Can cause low blood sugar reactions that last for many days. Rarely cause abnormal liver tests.
Meglitinides	repaglinide nateglinide	Prandin Starlix	Yes, but usually more mild than SAs	Side effects are rare and mild.
Biguanides	metformin	Glucophage Glucophage XR	Not usually	Often causes nausea, diarrhea. Don't use if kidneys or liver isn't normal. Don't use if you have congestive heart failure.

Glitazones	pioglitazone rosiglitazone	Actos Avandia	No	Don't use if liver problems or congestive heart failure; check liver tests periodically during the first year. Swelling (edema) of the feet and ankles most common side effect.
Alpha-glucosidase inhibitors (AGIs)	acarbose miglitol	Precose Glyset	No	Flatulence common. Don't use if kidneys or liver not normal or if history of bowel obstruction.

DRUGS THAT INCREASE INSULIN SECRETION

Sulfonylurea Agents

When I was learning about treating diabetes in 1980, sulfonylurea agents were the only type of oral medication available for treating type 2 diabetes. These drugs work to lower blood sugar levels, but are not my first choice for treating type 2 diabetes anymore. They stimulate the pancreas to increase the release of insulin into the bloodstream. I prefer the other, more "holistic" way to treat type 2 diabetes, which is to lower insulin resistance through diet and exercise. One problem with taking medication to increase insulin levels is that blood sugar levels can fall too low on a regular basis. This is especially problematic if a patient is trying to cut back on calories and increase exercise. Another consideration with using these drugs is weight gain; patients taking these pills report feeling hungrier. Some of the newer sulfonylurea agents, such as Amaryl, may have alleviated this concern.

I do have many patients who take these drugs. They seem to work more quickly than any of the other pills used for treating diabetes. Within a week or two of starting on sulfonylurea pills, blood sugar levels will be noticeably lower. Even diabetes patients taking other medications to stimulate insulin production may need a boost from a sulfonylurea agent. On the negative side, these drugs can cause frequent low blood sugar reactions. If this problem develops, the dose may have to be reduced.

Meglitinides

Prandin (repaglinide) and Starlix (nateglinide) are similar to the sulfonylurea agents in that they work to make the pancreas produce more insulin. However, the beauty of Prandin and Starlix is that they are short-acting and can be used to produce insulin to cover one meal at a time. This reduces some of the longer-term effects of increasing insulin levels: hunger and the risk for low blood sugar levels in the middle of the day. I find such drugs useful because they help me target exactly the kind of control a patient needs. For example, say a patient has great blood sugar levels after breakfast and lunch, but the levels are too high after dinner. By recommending the patient take Prandin or Starlix just before dinner, those after-dinner blood sugar levels can be lowered. In essence, it allows us to target just that one meal. Once on these drugs for a while, patients become quite good at adjusting their dose to match the meal. If a healthy, low-carb meal is eaten, the medication can be skipped. You also can skip the pill if you skip a meal, although missing meals is not a good idea. If you are celebrating your birthday or eating a meal containing extra carbohydrates, you can adjust to a higher dose of Prandin or Starlix.

The problem with such flexibility and control is that you have to remember to follow the plan.

I like for my patients to have this kind of flexibility. It allows them to make choices about their medication and diet. They are in control of their sugar balance. The problem with such flexibility and control is that you have to remember to follow the plan. We all know that it is much more difficult to take a pill several times per day than it is to take a pill once a day. I know for myself that I can remember to take pills when I brush my teeth, which is generally first thing in the morning and the last thing before bed. If I have to take pills in the middle of the day, I almost always forget. Studies done on patients to see how often they take pills have shown that the more often you have to take a pill the more likely you are to forget it. Using short-acting medication like Starlix or Prandin requires a commitment to remembering to take it when you need it (as well as having the experience to know when *not* to take it). The Prandin manufacturers make a little pill container that you can attach to your keychain so you always have your pills with you. This seems to help my patients, especially men. Women who carry purses usually can fit a bottle of pills somewhere inside. However, you do need to be sure you have the medication with you to take before you eat. Starlix and Prandin can be dangerous to take after you eat (they can drop blood sugar too low). They only work correctly if taken just before a meal, and are not the kind of medications that allow you to make up for missed doses.

DRUGS THAT LOWER INSULIN RESISTANCE

Metformin

Metformin only was introduced in the United States in the mid 1990s, although it had been used worldwide since 1957. This class of drugs actually dates back to medieval times. The active ingredient was found in a plant called french lilac or goat's rue and was used as an herbal medicine to treat people with symptoms of diabetes long before anyone knew what diabetes was.

Metformin's long history makes it a drug we know well in terms of risks and benefits. Interestingly, no one has ever figured out exactly how it works. We know that it doesn't increase insulin levels. It is thought that it works mostly by decreasing the amount of sugar your liver makes overnight. This action causes prebreakfast or fasting blood sugar levels to be lower, which improves blood sugar levels throughout the day. Metformin may also have a small effect on lowering insulin resistance, so the insulin your body produces works more effectively. In addition to lowering blood sugar levels, metformin may lower your risk of having a heart attack.

I have used metformin without a problem in hundreds and hundreds of patients.

I often select metformin as one of the first drugs I use for treating newly diagnosed type 2 diabetes. However, there are very specific guidelines for using metformin and patients must fit the criteria in order for it to be prescribed. Otherwise (as I will discuss), you put yourself at risk for a severe, harmful side effect. I have used metformin without a problem in hundreds and hundreds of patients. Used with care within a select group, metformin usually is my drug treatment of choice.

Metformin is notable for being the only effective diabetes drug that doesn't cause weight gain. This is probably because taking it makes you feel a little sick to your stomach, and therefore less hungry. As your appetite decreases slightly, your blood sugar levels improve. But metformin is *not* a weight loss drug, although if you do go on a low-calorie diet while taking it, metformin will not cause low blood sugar reactions.

The downside to metformin is that it often causes side effects in the intestinal system. Some patients mention feeling nauseated, bloated, and having diarrhea. It almost always changes people's bowel habits; the drug is stored in your small intestine so it alters how your intestines process food. Metformin can cause such bad diarrhea that the drug's use must be stopped. I've had patients who were taking it go see their primary care doctors and have extensive testing done for gastric problems. When I hear about this I usually say, "There's nothing wrong with your insides. Just stop the metformin and you'll feel fine." Usually, I'm right. However, there are things you can do to make this reaction less intense. You should always take metformin with food in your stomach to buffer any negative reaction. Taking metformin at dinnertime makes sense because it is at its strongest overnight. That way, if you do have a reaction, at least you will most likely be at home. There is also a new form of metformin, called Glucophage XR, that is longer-acting and may cause fewer problems.

> **You should always take metformin with food in your stomach to buffer any negative reaction.**

I usually start patients off with a low dose, usually 500 mg, and increase the dose every two weeks if their systems tolerate it. If they feel okay after that (or only experience a little diarrhea or queasiness the first day or two), I have them increase the metformin dose to two 500 mg tablets with dinner. At that point I schedule a clinic visit to check progress and blood sugar levels. If all is well, I increase the dose to one 500 mg pill in the morning and the two pills at dinner. This 1,500-mg-per-day dose is often the amount of metformin necessary to control blood sugar levels. You can go up to 2,000 mg (two pills in the morning and two in the evening), but that's generally the limit. I often can't get patients to take more than 1,500 mg per day, due to the side effects. Yet, metformin is such a good, reliable drug that I feel it is worth working through the side effects if possible, to get the dose right.

A more serious side effect of metformin is lactic acidosis. This means that acid builds up in your blood. If this rare event happens to you, there is a 50/50 chance that you will die. You can minimize the chance of this problem if you know what to watch for. First, the FDA has very strict rules that doctors are supposed to follow before they start you on metformin. Can you be certain you doctor is following these rules? Unfortunately, the answer is no. I have seen many patients taking metformin who shouldn't have been on it. Fortunately, they all were fine, but it put them at risk for trouble in the future.

You probably should double-check your lab results yourself, and make sure you qualify to take the drug safely. Your kidneys must be working normally. This means that the blood test for your kidney function (the creatinine level) comes back normal. This creatinine level should be less than 1.4 if you are female and less than 1.5 if you are male.

Patients who have, or are prone to, congestive heart failure (when the heart doesn't pump blood efficiently) should be screened out. Prior liver damage is another concern, as is drinking excessive amounts of alcohol (a little bit of alcohol is okay). You're not a metformin candidate, either, if you have chronic lung disease that reduces your oxygen supply. Metformin won't hurt healthy kidneys, liver, or heart, but metformin users should have them tested every six months. If these organs already are damaged, metformin can build up in your system and cause a bad reaction. What it comes down to is: if you are chronically ill in some way you shouldn't take metformin. And metformin shouldn't be taken if there is any sudden serious change in your health. Examples would be a car accident, or if you were in the hospital for a procedure, or needed to have a test done that required dye to be injected into your veins. In cases like this, I tell patients not to resume taking metformin until they are completely recovered and we have tested their kidneys to make sure they are functioning properly.

Do's and Don'ts for Taking Metformin

- Do take it with food.

- Do increase the dose slowly.

- Do tell your doctor if you have diarrhea or nausea.

- Do stop taking it if you are having a test where dye will be injected into your veins.

- Do make sure you have your kidneys and liver tested regularly.

- Don't take it if your kidneys aren't normal.

- Don't take it if your liver isn't nearly normal.

- Don't take it if you have congestive heart failure.

- Don't take it if you drink more than two glasses of alcohol per day.

- Don't take it if you are sick or in the the hospital.

- Don't be needlessly afraid. This is a good drug.

Glitazones (Actos and Avandia)

In 1997 Rezulin, the first of a new class of drug called glitazones, came on the market. You may recall the storm of media attention this drug received. After lots of politics and the raising of some real health concerns, Rezulin was pulled off the market. It has since been replaced by Actos and Avandia, two other drugs in the glitazone family. As in all families, these related glitazone drugs are very similar, yet have distinct differences.

I participated in one of the preliminary Rezulin clinical trial sites when I was at UCLA. This allowed me to understand the drug first-hand and be part of the small group that shared information on the trials. I was initially a supporter of Rezulin. But like all drugs, it had its risks and benefits. I'll tell you more about Rezulin in a moment.

The drugs mentioned above have extended names within the glitazone family—Rezulin is tro*glitazone,* Actos is pio*glitazone,* and Avandia is rosi*glitazone.* They also have an even longer scientific name: thiazolidinediones (TZDs). The main effect of glitazones is to lower insulin resistance in the same way that exercise and weight loss do. Sometimes I call these drugs "exercise in a pill." They treat type 2 diabetes by making you more sensitive to the insulin you produce. We are starting to see indications that the glitazones have an even greater benefit beyond lowering insulin resistance. Research suggests that they may not only stimulate the pancreas to continue making insulin (instead of burning out, as with other oral medications), but may possibly lower the risk of heart attack and stroke. There are many big studies under way systematically reviewing the potential benefits of glitazones. But the results so far, from my experience and that of my colleagues in clinical research, have been positive. The *right patients* seem to do much better than expected on these medications.

Sometimes I call these drugs "exercise in a pill."

The Rezulin Story

So what happened with the first drug, Rezulin? Though it was a promising new treatment option, it was found to cause liver damage in a small group of patients. The active ingredients were bound to vitamin E to make the drug safer, but this assumption proved fatally wrong. Though rare, the liver damage could be so severe patients died from it.

Two new glitazones came on the market after Rezulin, each designed to offer a different approach. Actos and Avandia are not attached to vitamin E and don't cause liver damage in the same way Rezulin did. However, because their relative, Rezulin, caused liver damage, it still is recommended (though no longer FDA-required) that regular liver tests be performed on patients taking them.

Because I do research with new medications, I know how often we are asked to monitor blood tests when working with new drugs. I also know that when a new drug is approved by the FDA it is often tested in only five thousand or so people. Because some side effects occur in one out of fifty thousand people, these side effects are unknown until a drug is on the market for a year or more. Therefore, whenever I prescribe a recently released drug for a patient, I monitor extra carefully, checking liver, kidneys, and blood count every two to three months to be sure no problems develop. When I first used Rezulin, I checked liver functions every other month in my patients, as I do with any new class of medication. And although an occasional patient had a slight increase in liver tests, none had serious problems.

Obviously, you need to know whether your doctor is giving you a new drug or one that has been on the market for a while. You need to read the patient package insert to learn about side effects and blood testing requirements. This kind of awareness allows use of medications in the safest way possible, enhancing their benefits and lowering their risks.

You need to know whether your doctor is giving you a new drug or one that has been on the market for a while.

Using Actos and Avandia

Any time a person with type 2 diabetes becomes less resistant to the effects of insulin, blood sugar levels come down. The better drugs, including Actos and Avandia, do this without causing blood sugar to drop too low. Actos is taken just once a day. Avandia is taken either once or twice a day. Both drugs have relatively few side effects, but there are some things about them you need to know. Your liver tests should be normal or near normal to start on one of these medications and your liver should be tested periodically (maybe once every three to six months for the first year). If your liver tests increase while taking one of these drugs, you should stop. I have never seen a liver problem that I thought was caused by either Actos or Avandia, but I still recommend having liver tests done regularly to be sure things are still normal.

There is a common, generally minor, side effect from taking Actos or Avandia: edema, or swollen ankles. The swelling is usually slight and nothing to worry about. (Many overweight people without diabetes have some ankle swelling.) But sometimes the swelling is more severe and it means that the medication should be stopped. We don't understand why these drugs can cause swelling, but, ironically, it may be related to one of their benefits. Both these glitazones may relax blood vessels and lower blood pressure (help-ing your heart). At the same time, the drugs may cause blood ves-sels to become more permeable to water, allowing a little fluid to leak out and potentially to pool in the extremities.

***Both these drugs make your body
use insulin more efficiently.***

The swelling that results only becomes serious if you have con-gestive heart failure, a condition in which the heart isn't pumping well enough. Two of the symptoms of congestive heart failure are shortness of breath when walking, especially uphill, and needing to sleep propped up on pillows at night (because sleeping flat would cause you to feel very short of breath). The more fluid in your body, the harder the heart has to work. If your heart already doesn't pump efficiently, the excess fluid can leak into more dan-gerous places than the ankles, such as the lungs. In people with-out congestive heart failure (who may have some heart damage they possibly don't know about) extra fluid can tip them into con-gestive heart failure. Both congestive heart failure and fluid in the lungs are common problems in people with poorly controlled or late-diagnosed diabetes.

The rules, then, of using Actos and Avandia are simple: Don't take them if your liver isn't normal or if you have congestive heart failure. One other caution is to eat less to avoid gaining weight once your blood sugars get better. Both these drugs make your body use insulin more efficiently. As this happens, your body will begin to store, as fat, the extra calories you are receiving. People who don't change their diets normally will gain 5 to 10 pounds on these drugs. If there is a positive to this, it's that the new fat is dis-tributed throughout your body, not just in your center where fat is a greater problem. It can be discouraging for patients to *gain* weight when they have a disease that is supposed to be treated by weight loss. But you can lose the weight after you start on a glitazone if you put your mind to it.

I tend to prescribe Actos more than Avandia, because the ef-fects on triglyceride and cholesterol levels are better with Actos, but the acclimating process is similar with both drugs. I start patients out with a very small dose of Actos—15 mg once a day—to lessen the risk for side effects. It can be taken with or without food, in the morning or the evening. Watch for swelling in your feet or shortness of breath. Don't expect to see any real fall in blood sugar levels early on, because 15 mg is such a tiny dose and these pills take twelve to sixteen weeks to fully work. After one month, if there are no problems, the dosage is increased from 15 mg to 30 mg. I ask patients newly on glitazones to come back to see me after a total of three months to have a liver test. Then, in most cases, patients stay on the 30-mg dose for another month or two as blood sugar levels are closely monitored. I recommend checking your liver every three months for that first year. If more Actos is needed, the dosage can be increased to 45 mg, but often I see a satisfactory response at 30 mg and stay with it.

Do's and Don'ts for Taking Glitazones

- Do take them at any time of day you'll remember, with or without food.

- Do have your liver tested before you start and every three to six months for the first year. Call your doctor if you develop swelling in your legs or shortness of breath.

- Do eat slightly less so you don't gain weight.

- Don't take them if your liver is not normal.

- Don't take them if you have congestive heart failure.

- Don't take them if you have swelling in your legs.

- Don't expect a rapid fall in your blood sugars.

DRUGS THAT LIMIT GLUCOSE ABSORPTION

Alpha-Glucosidase Inhibitors (Precose and Glyset)

Why wait to talk about these "wonder drugs" last? It seems like a dream, to treat diabetes by decreasing the amount of carbohydrate that is absorbed in the intestines. This would be an ideal way to lower blood sugar levels and weight at the same time. Unfortunately, it's still a dream; we're not there quite yet.

Alpha-glucosidase inhibitors (AGIs) do lower your blood sugar increase after eating. But they only improve blood sugar control by a very small amount (for example, bringing your fasting blood sugar from 200 mg/dl to 180, instead of down to 90–130). They frequently cause unpleasant side effects, too, the most common being the production of large amounts of intestinal gas. I think you get the picture.

My patients who have tried these drugs find that the social embarrassment level is so high that they either won't go out in public or stop taking the drug when out in public. European studies using higher doses seem to get better results. But in my practice I hardly ever use them, partly because my patients need a greater improvement in their blood sugar levels than these drugs can bring about. Certainly, I wouldn't stop someone from taking one of these drugs if the person were already on them, and I would prescribe the drugs if asked.

If you are going to take alpha-glucosidase inhibitors, your doctor needs to be sure that your kidneys are normal (although not as normal as with metformin—in this case, a creatinine level of less than 2 mg/dl is considered okay); your liver is normal; and you haven't had problems with bowel obstructions or other problems with your gut. Patients start by taking a very small dose, usually 25 mg, before each meal. The drug, as I explained, lowers the amount of carbohydrate your body absorbs. These pills won't do much if you don't eat much carbohydrate. But if you eat a plateful of pasta, it will cut back on how much carbohydrate goes into your bloodstream as sugar. Usually there is not much effect at the lowest dose, but you can increase the amount you take gradually, as your gut adjusts. The voluminous gas is caused by the undigested carbohydrate that flows to your colon. The carbohydrates mix with bacteria that live in the colon and a great fermentation process begins. This fermentation produces the gas.

One important note: If you take these drugs, along with reducing carbohydrate uptake, they may alter how quickly your body can absorb sugar when treating a low blood sugar reaction. These drugs don't cause low blood sugar reactions all by themselves, but if you take them along with a drug that does (such as glyburide or insulin), your blood sugar levels could fall and you would need to treat reactions with glucose tablets or milk, not table sugar.

GUT HORMONES

These drugs are under development and some, if not all, of them will be available for treating diabetes. They are released from your gut and affect digestion, blood sugar levels, appetite, weight, and production of beta cells (the cells that make insulin). Ideally these drugs will help with weight loss at the same time they lower blood sugar levels. I am looking forward to having these agents available to add to our repertoire for treating both type 1 and type 2 diabetes.

HERBAL AND ALTERNATIVE APPROACHES FOR TREATING TYPE 2 DIABETES

Almost every week, it seems, something new is introduced as the great new breakthrough for treating diabetes. I have seen so many new herbal or weight loss compounds come and go, most quietly touting a side benefit of improving diabetes control. I have worked with doctors who practice Eastern medicine and acupuncture, and who use traditional herbal therapies. They tell me that although their herbs may help lower the risk for complications of diabetes, they don't lower blood sugar levels much. I'm all for a patient trying a new preparation for treating diabetes. But I've never seen gymnema sylvestre, bitter melon, pancreas tonic, vanadium, chromium, or any of the other alternative diabetes treatments work in a lasting way, although some may cause a slight blood sugar reduction.

One of the reasons, I think, that so many herbalists can claim success is that they don't do controlled studies with their drugs. They don't, for example, compare their drug/supplement/elixir to a sugar pill placebo. And in clinical diabetes studies there is a huge response rate to the placebos. It is not uncommon for there to be a 20 to 30 percent improvement in blood sugars when study participants are told they are taking a miracle drug for their diabetes. Perhaps it is because they suddenly start exercising more or watching what they eat (because they are in a research study). Personally, I don't mind this placebo effect if it means that people are healthier. If only the results could be sustained over time.

Although herbs may help lower the risk for complications of diabetes, they don't lower blood sugar levels.

One of the few supplements shown to be helpful in diabetes is cinnamon—about ½ teaspoonful taken with each meal. As soon as this story came out in the newspaper, approximately half of my patients began adding cinnamon to their meals. Have I seen much improvement in their blood sugars? A little bit . . . in a few. And if you like cinnamon, it probably couldn't hurt. Just don't spend lots of money on herbal preparations unless they really seem to be making a big difference in your blood sugar or cholesterol levels. And be sure to bring whatever you're taking in to your doctor, so he or she can note what they are. Herbal or not, they are still medications and can potentially interact with other drugs you are taking.

MY APPROACH TO THE USE OF PILLS WHEN TREATING TYPE 2 DIABETES

Now that you are familiar with all of the tools for treating type 2 diabetes, I want to share with you how I use them. I wish I could always be successful at treating diabetes with just nutrition and exercise, but that just doesn't happen in every case. None of us likes to take pills, but neither pills nor western medicine is the enemy. For many people the benefits of medication far outweigh the risks. This is not to say that taking pills is without risk. Any pill you take, whether it is a natural herbal medicine, a Tylenol tablet, or a drug for lowering your blood sugar levels, carries a risk. Understanding the expected risk from each medication *as well as* the benefit is the key.

But having diabetes is a risky disease. Not treating it causes complications that seem every bit as bad to me as watching someone die from cancer. Treatment usually requires not one or two different medications, but nine or ten, each acting together to control the disease. I think that someday we may have one or two pills that do the work of ten, but today we have to use what works.

Understanding the expected risk from each medication as well as the benefit is the key.

When I prescribe any new medicine to a patient, I always give my risk and benefit lecture. I explain why I have chosen a particular pill for them, what I expect as a benefit, and what I have done (and will continue to do) to minimize any risk. If you come to see me and we decide you need to start on an oral medication to lower your blood sugar levels, chances are I'll start with either metformin or a glitazone (Actos or Avandia) if your blood sugar levels are lower than 300. My two main goals are to lower your blood sugar levels and help reduce your risk of heart disease. The ultimate goal, of course, is to help you avoid diabetic complications.

I know that none of these drugs will cause you to have low blood sugar reactions (hypoglycemia). Metformin may help you with weight loss and I know that the glitazones, when used alone, won't cause much weight gain (which is reversible with a little effort). I also know that both of the glitazones will help raise your good (HDL) cholesterol level, although Actos may lower your triglyceride levels more than Avandia does.

Let's say that on your first visit you described the classic symptoms of excessive thirst, weight loss, and very high blood sugar levels (over 300). I would start you immediately on a big dose of a sulfonylurea agent. This class of drugs works rapidly and could help bring your blood sugar levels down in a matter of days. Some doctors start insulin in this situation, but I like to give people the chance to succeed on oral medications first. For people who respond to this treatment, I then slowly lower the dose of the sulfonylurea agent and start the shift to metformin and/or a glitazone.

Metformin, glitazones, and sulfonylurea agents all will lower blood sugar levels by about the same amount, although they do it differently. I prefer to use metformin and glitazones for continuing care because I have found that more patients experience low blood sugar reactions on sulfonylurea agents. This was especially true when patients were doing the right thing and cutting back on calories and exercising more. Sometimes people on sulfonylurea agents have to eat more to counteract hypoglycemia and, consequently, they gain weight. This can discourage them as they work to make lasting lifestyle changes.

I prefer to use metformin and glitazones for continuing care because I have found that more patients experience low blood sugar reactions on sulfonylurea agents.

My preferred approach is based on experience with these newer drugs, and the benefits I believe they have. Sulfonylurea agents still have a place. They have been around since 1940 and cost only pennies a day. Sulfonylurea agents also can be used for almost anyone—you don't have to worry unduly about your kidney or liver functions, or if you have congestive heart failure. If your doctor wants you to try this type of drug first, just watch out for low blood sugar reactions. You may need to cut back on the dose if you start seriously cutting calories and increasing exercise.

When I give lectures to doctors, I tell them that the first choice of therapy, while important, is probably not the ultimate answer. Most of their patients will end up taking two or more medications for their diabetes. Approaches vary and often a doctor's choices are limited by his or her medical system. Some insurance plans and medical groups insist on following a specified order when it comes to prescribing medications so doctors don't jump to the newer, more expensive medications without giving the old ones a chance. This is a reasonable attempt at controlling health care costs. But I also like to teach doctors what I would do, without the restrictions.

Most of their patients will end up taking two or more medications for their diabetes.

When a single medication isn't enough, my next step is to prescribe the combination of metformin plus a glitazone. The metformin cuts down the weight gain of the glitazone and the two work together well to control type 2 diabetes. Again, neither will cause frequent low blood sugar reactions and both are likely to lower the risk for heart disease. If you are taking a sulfonylurea agent and need to add a second medication, I would probably add metformin. Adding a glitazone could also be an option.

When two drugs do not provide enough control, a patient may need something to increase the amount of insulin production. An after-dinner blood test can tell us if it is time to add a third medication. If blood sugars go up significantly just after a meal, I add Prandin or Starlix. Taken before eating, these target that postprandial high blood sugar. If, on the other hand, a patient has high levels nearly all the time, I would probably add in a small dose of a sulfonylurea agent. Some doctors would just have you take insulin when more than two medications are called for. I usually wait until we try three oral medications. I'm not opposed to insulin shots, but most people prefer pills to shots.

Sometimes patients' choices and combinations are limited by side effects or any conditions they might have (such as kidney or liver damage) that preclude the use of one drug or another. Cost also is an issue, particularly if you (and not insurance) are paying for your medications. The glitazones are by far the most expensive oral diabetes drugs. Metformin and sulfonylurea agents are available as low-cost generics. Again, there is no one best or set way to treat type 2 diabetes. Each patient and health care plan is different. Individual doctors have their own treatment experience and their options may be dictated by a practice.

Medication and Blood Sugar Monitoring

Every patient needs to ask the following questions when starting medication: Why am I taking this drug? What is it supposed to do? How do I know the drug is doing its job? and What should I be monitoring to be sure this drug is safe? Diabetes gives us big clues to these answers in the form of blood sugar levels. You can monitor your blood sugar levels with a glucose meter at home to make sure that your blood sugar levels before meals are regularly in the 90 to 130 md/dl range, and that two hours after eating your blood sugar levels are less than 180. Normal blood sugar levels are even lower: 70 to 110 before meals and less than 140 after eating.

Patients who test at home should take their meters or logs to provider visits. This provides a snapshot of your current diabetes situation and can help doctors make decisions based on recent, cumulative data. The figures from testing first thing in the morning, and then two hours after a meal, are usually most helpful. Not every doctor recommends that people with type 2 diabetes test blood sugar levels at home. If you're feeling stable and are not changing lifestyle or medication, you probably don't need to. But if you are sick or adjusting your medication, it's good to know what is happening to your blood sugar numbers.

The figures from testing first thing in the morning, and then two hours after a meal, are usually most helpful.

Using medication, we attempt to match normal blood sugar levels without having them fall too low. Low blood sugars occur mostly with drugs that increase insulin secretion, such as sulfonylurea agents, or with insulin shots. Mild low blood sugar reactions, ones that you can sense and can easily treat, are not a serious health risk, although they can be uncomfortable and scary. Low blood sugar reactions cause people to feel unusually weak, shaky, hungry, and sweaty. The symptoms go away as soon as you have 15 grams of rapid-acting sugar in the form of either juice, raisins or dates, nondiet soda, candy, or glucose tablets. For reactions that don't go away easily, you may need to go to the emergency room to be given sugar intravenously. (For more on hypoglycemia see chapter 5 and pages 269–272 in chapter 15.)

**The overall goal is to help patients have blood sugars
as close to normal as possible, without incurring
low blood sugar reactions.**

The overall goal is to help patients have blood sugars as close to normal as possible, without incurring low blood sugar reactions. It's a fine line to walk, which is why I like the combination of metformin and a glitazone that rarely drops levels too low. When blood sugar levels are in the range of 90 to 130 mg/dl before meals and less than 180 after, blood sugar control will show as less than 7 percent on an A1C test. If A1C level rises above 7 percent, the addition of another medication needs to be considered. By having the A1C level measured every three months you can tell if you are deviating from this goal. If starting a new medication doesn't keep your A1C less than 7 percent, the medication probably needs to be changed or dosage increased. *Check with your physician before changing any medication on your own.* In some cases, particularly with the glitazones, it may take several weeks to see an initial response.

Is Using Multiple Drugs Safe?

All of these drugs used in type 2 diabetes work together and interact without problems. Metformin and either of the glitazones, for example, are complementary in their actions. Both can also be safely combined with a sulfonylurea agent, plus either Prandin or Starlix. Insulin, too, can be used with any of these pills.

Along with any of the medications mentioned above, you can and probably should be taking the following additional drugs to keep your heart healthy: aspirin, a statin to lower cholesterol, a fibrate to lower triglycerides, and an ACE inhibitor and/or ARB to lower blood pressure. Ask your doctor.

Combination Pills

So now maybe you're asking this perfectly reasonable question: If you have to take all these different pills and the drugs interact

TABLE 12. SAFE MONITORING OF DIABETES MEDICATION

Drug	Test	How Often	When to Worry
Sulfonylurea agent (e.g., glyburide, Glucotrol, or Amaryl)	None needed		
Meglitinide (Prandin or Starlix)	None needed		
Metformin	Creatinine (kidney)	One or twice a year—more often if it is borderline high	Stop metformin if creatinine is 1.4 mg/dl or greater in a female, 1.5 or greater in a male
Metformin	ALT and AST (liver), CBC (blood count)	Once a year	Stop metformin if serious liver abnormalities; measure vitamin B_{12} levels if anemic
Glitazone	ALT, AST (liver)	Every three to six months for the first year	Stop the glitazone if the ALT or AST rises above normal (you need to ask your health care provider for help in interpreting this)

well, why not just mix the various medications into one single pill? Combination pills that contain two different drugs do exist, but I don't recommend them. Though most of us prefer taking fewer pills, I have found in my experience that single-purpose medications provide greater control and more measurable results. If, for example, you were to start taking a metformin and glyburide combination pill (there's one available called Glucovance) and you began having diarrhea, you would stop taking the pill and, therefore, you'd be stopping *all* of your diabetes medication. Not a good idea. But if you were on metformin and glyburide separately and had the same reaction, you would instead just cut back or stop the metformin, leaving the glyburide to control your blood sugar levels. Here's another illustration. If you were taking the Glucovance combination and your blood sugar levels fell too low, we would have to lower the dosage. This would cut back on both the metformin and the glyburide you were taking, when the proper approach would be to lower only the dose of glyburide and not the metformin. Almost none of my patients are on fixed combination pills for their diabetes. In my experience it works out better to be able to individually adjust medication dosage, raising or lowering each dose freely, without the constraint of a prefixed drug formulation. However, if you are stable on two pills and a combination dose pill with the same ingredients is available, you may wish to switch to reduce the number of pills you are taking.

All the medications mentioned above are effective treatments for type 2 diabetes. But sometimes blood sugar levels stay stubbornly high. When that happens there is only one reliable drug to use—the body's own solution to the problem, insulin.

In my experience it works out better to be able to individually adjust medication dosage, raising or lowering each dose freely, without the constraint of a prefixed drug formulation.

TWELVE

THE ART OF USING INSULIN

THE SCARIEST DRUG OF ALL

No other drug that I prescribe makes people more nervous than insulin. Fear of needles is part of it, but it's not just that. Other injectable therapies don't seem to frighten patients as much, even growth hormone with its significant potential side effects. Some fear of insulin is justified—it's a powerful hormone—and some is based on misconception. These are the five main reasons people fear it: (1) they fear insulin will cause their health to get worse; (2) they fear becoming addicted to an injectable drug; (3) they fear the pain of needle puncture; (4) they fear having to completely change their lifestyle; and (5) they fear they have failed in their treatment. All of these are valid concerns and in each case understanding insulin, what it means, what it does, why it is sometimes necessary, and how it can seamlessly fit into your lifestyle will help address your fears. Let's take a closer look at each of these five fears.

Insulin is part of the solution, not the problem.

Fear #1: My Health Will Deteriorate

At least once a week, when I am discussing starting insulin with a patient, I hear a story like, "My aunt Trudy started taking insulin shots and one month later went blind," or "My grandfather went on insulin and they had to cut off his leg." Of course, these events happened, and they were hell on the people who endured them and painful to their loved ones, my patients, who were helpless witnesses. But insulin didn't *cause* these things to happen. Unfortunately, they would have happened anyway, likely because by the time Aunt Trudy's or Grandpa's physicians realized the extent to which diabetes complications had overtaken their health and prescribed the insulin, it was too late. It takes ten to twenty years to build up the damage that leads to blindness and amputation. That means years of having blood sugars that are too high and the resultant clogging of the arteries that lead to the eyes or the legs, causing the tissue to die from decreased blood flow. Starting insulin late in the disease's course neither prevents nor reverses damage that has already been done. The reason you *want* to start insulin as soon as it is necessary is to avoid *ever* having such complications. Insulin is part of the solution, not the problem.

Fear #2: I Don't Want to Become Addicted

Many patients express concern about addiction or about becoming dependent on insulin in a negative way. They've seen pictures or images of heroin addicts "shooting up" and somehow think that using insulin is the same. Insulin couldn't be more different. It is a hormone—something your body makes naturally (like estrogen, testosterone, and thyroid hormone) and it's legal. The reason you need insulin injections is simply because your body has stopped making enough insulin on its own. You must supplement what is missing. You don't become addicted to insulin! You can stop using it anytime. But if you don't give yourself a scheduled shot, your blood sugars will go up. It is as simple as that. There's no drug "withdrawal" involved.

(Please note: Stopping the use of insulin when you have type 1 diabetes is another story altogether. In type 1, the pancreas is damaged to the point where it makes no insulin whatsoever. Insulin in patients with type 1 diabetes is therefore essential to life.)

My best advice if you have type 2 diabetes and are fearful of becoming addicted to insulin shots is to lose weight and increase your physical activity. Then you can stop your insulin injections safely, without fear of blood sugar repercussions.

Fear #3: Insulin Shots Hurt

One of my diabetes doctor friends requires all of his patients to give themselves a saline shot the very first day he meets them, whether or not they require insulin at this time. He does this so they know from the get-go not to be afraid even if they are many years away from needing insulin. I think this is a great way of fending off the fear, because patients soon realize that insulin shots don't really hurt all that much. I won't lie; they aren't painless, and occasionally they sting if you hit a nerve bundle. Most of my long-time patients tell me they don't even feel the shots anymore.

A couple of other points (no pun intended): When you inject insulin, you inject into fatty tissue. This hurts less than injecting into muscle. Finally, there are injectors available on the market that can reduce pain, as can using syringes with the smallest needle gauge. There's more about all this in chapter 15.

Fear #4: Insulin Will Completely Change My Lifestyle

Years ago, taking insulin often meant conforming to a fairly strict schedule, which, I will admit, was a pain. Now there are better, newer insulins that can be matched to your lifestyle rather than the other way around. Most of my type 2 patients are able to continue on pills during the day (to treat the insulin resistance) and give an injection only once a day. This way, the insulin works overnight to lower the fasting blood sugar level and the pills work during the day. Most people find that they can give one shot a day without any change at all to their lifestyle. It's much less of a hassle having to do it at night away from the workplace and the demands of the day. Also, if these patients ever have to give themselves more shots, they are used to it and it's not as big a deal.

Fear #5: I Need Insulin Because I Have Failed at Treating My Diabetes

Diabetes is a disease that, in most cases, gets worse over time. Many people need to start insulin injections because their body has stopped making enough insulin to keep their blood sugar levels normal, in spite of any oral medications and lifestyle changes. Not everyone ends up needing insulin, of course, but many do. And it isn't their fault; it isn't a failure on their part to manage their diabetes. It is the nature of the disease. We don't say that someone has "failed" when they need their appendix taken out or when antibiotics are required for treating pneumonia or when they take a pill for a migraine.

Many physicians hold out insulin shots as a threat. They tell their patients, "If you don't lose weight, you'll need to start on insulin." Suddenly, insulin is seen as a punishment, a sign of inadequacy. The fact is, insulin is simply another treatment for your diabetes, another tool to help you keep your blood sugar levels in the normal range. The goal is to avoid developing the complications of diabetes. In a way, it doesn't matter which tools you need to accomplish this—whether it is through lifestyle or pills or insulin or all three. Insulin is a means to an end. And in this case the end is a new beginning.

WHAT IS INSULIN?

Insulin is a naturally occurring hormone that is made by the beta cells in the human pancreas. Dogs, cows, pigs, and fish all make insulin, as well. Scientists discovered they could treat diabetes by grinding up a dog pancreas and injecting it into a dog. The first insulin used in humans was from a cow. For many years (including when I first became a doctor in 1983), the insulin that was used in humans came from cows or pigs. About fifteen years ago, scientists mastered synthetic human insulin; all of the insulin administered to humans today is made in a laboratory.

Insulin shots mimic the normal release of insulin from the pancreas. Someone giving themselves insulin injections is, in essence, acting as their own pancreas, doing consciously what the body does reflexively. Synthetic insulin is formulated to work over a set period of time—anywhere from very fast to very slowly. Some insulin has a peak—a fairly predictable time after injection when we expect it to work most strongly. NPH insulin, for instance, is called intermediate-acting insulin. It starts working four to six hours after it is given and then peaks in ten to twelve hours. The total time it lasts in the body is about twenty-four hours.

There are many more types of insulin, which will be discussed in chapter 15.

Most people with type 2 diabetes who need insulin use intermediate-acting NPH insulin and/or a long-acting type. The available long-acting insulin is called glargine (Lantus) [detemir (Levemir is under development)]. Lantus insulin works slowly in the body over about twenty-four hours and don't have much of a peak. This makes its action more steady and predictable. These relatively new insulins have been altered slightly to make them absorb more slowly than other kinds in order to more closely match the slow release of natural insulin from the pancreas of a person without diabetes. Other insulins include short acting regular and rapid acting aspart (Novolog) and lispro (Humalog) which are given before meals.

If you need to begin taking insulin, this book can help. But you also will need a teacher, either a diabetes educator or your doctor. You'll need to learn the specifics about the type of insulin you'll be using and how it will affect your body from the beginning, which only your educator or doctor can provide. You need to be taught how to draw the correct amount of insulin up into the syringe, where and how to give the injection, and how to dispose of the needles. Usually you will need at least two lessons. The first is for learning the basic information and the second is for feedback and questions.

Novorapid

TABLE 13. BASIC TYPES OF INSULIN

Name	When Does It Start Working?	When Does It Act Most Strongly?	What Does It Look Like?	Can I Mix It with Other Insulin?
Humalog and Novolog (insulin analogues)	Immediately —you can give it right before you eat.	In 1 to 2 hours; and it lasts for about 4 hours.	Clear	Yes, except with Lantus.

Regular human insulin	This starts to work in 30 minutes so you need to use it 20 to 30 minutes before eating.	In 2 to 3 hours; and it lasts for about 6 hours.	Clear	Yes, except with Lantus.
NPH human insulin	It starts to act 4 to 6 hours after you inject it, so this insulin is given to have a delayed, not immediate, effect.	In 10 to 12 hours; and it lasts for 24 hours.	Cloudy	Yes, except with Lantus.
Lantus insulin (glargine)	Starts working slowly after injection; no real sudden action.	No peak. It lasts about 24 hours.	Clear	Do not mix this insulin with others.

Many people mistake Humulin and Novolin for *types* of insulin when actually they are brand names. Humulin is Lilly's brand of human insulin and can be either formulated as NPH or regular. Novolin is Novo Nordisk's brand of human insulin and it can also either be NPH or regular. What you need to know is the *type* of insulin you are taking. It's not enough to tell the pharmacist the brand name; you have to say whether the insulin is regular or NPH.

Insulin mixtures, which will be discussed shortly, are labeled by how much of what type of insulin is found in the mixture. So 70/30 usually means a ratio of 70 percent NPH and 30 percent regular, although it could mean 70 percent NPH and 30 percent Novolog. If you are ever in doubt as to what type of insulin you are taking, I recommend bringing your insulin bottles to your appointments so your health care provider knows exactly what you're taking and can review any test results accordingly. (Sometimes even pharmacists fill the prescriptions wrong—the types of insulin are increasing all the time and it is hard for health care providers, much less patients, to keep them all straight.) Check before you inject!

USING BEDTIME INSULIN/DAYTIME ORAL (BIDO) AGENTS

Here's a hypothetical patient: she has had high blood sugar levels (an A1C greater than 7 percent) despite taking the maximum of pills and making major efforts to change her diet and increase her exercise. In this case, I would start her on one shot of NPH (a cloudy, intermediate-acting insulin) or Lantus (a clear, long-acting insulin) at bedtime. Generally, I start patients like this on 10 to 12 "units" (an insulin measure) at bedtime and continue their daytime oral medications. The goal of the bedtime (or morning) insulin is to lower prebreakfast blood sugar to normal, around 100 mg/dl. It may ultimately take 40 to 50 units of insulin to bring a morning sugar level to this level. I start slowly, as above, to minimize the chance of a patient having an early low blood sugar reaction and becoming uncomfortable using insulin.

I ask patients to test their blood sugar level first thing in the morning and then again before dinner. That way, I can see how well balanced the effects of the insulin (given overnight) and the oral pills (taken in the daytime) are. If before-dinner blood sugar level drops too low, I decrease the dose of some of the pills (the ones that increase insulin secretion, like glyburide, glipizide, or Amaryl). If the morning blood sugar level falls too low, I decrease the dose of the bedtime insulin.

You shouldn't worry that giving a shot of insulin at bedtime will cause problems in the middle of the night. Your liver makes sugar all night long and the insulin shot balances the sugar your body makes. The reason I generally start patients with a low dose and go up gradually is because I want to see how their body reacts to the insulin.

Everyone is different—some people need only 10 units of insulin at bedtime while others need 100 units or so. The problem more often than not is giving someone *too little* insulin to bring the morning blood sugar level to normal.

If the blood sugar level before dinner doesn't fall, and remains above the premeal target of 90 to 130 mg/dl more than just one nightly shot of insulin is needed. But I have found that the one-shot-per-night approach can work, if there is frequent contact with the health care team and the insulin dose is slowly but surely increased each week until the morning blood sugar level is around 100. I also teach my patients to increase their own insulin dose by 2 to 4 units each week if their morning blood sugar level is above 150. *But don't do this on your own unless your physician or nurse educator suggests it.*

Everyone is different—some people need only 10 units of insulin at bedtime while others need 100 units or so.

Giving an injection before bedtime doesn't work for everyone. Some people, despite the best efforts of their doctors and educators, remain concerned about blood sugars becoming too low in the middle of the night, or they simply forget to inject before bed. If that's the case, an alternative approach is to take an injection of a long-acting insulin (such as Lantus) before breakfast. This will lower the morning blood sugar level because it lasts approximately twenty-four hours in the system, and it tends to cause fewer low sugar reactions in the middle of the night than a shot of NPH at bedtime. If you are having trouble reaching your goals on NPH you may want to ask your diabetes health care provider about switching to Lantus.

All these pills and insulins, and combinations of both, can be confusing. Just remember that the goal is to match the insulin production of a healthy pancreas. A normal pancreas will produce a base level of insulin throughout the day and increase production when you eat, keeping blood sugars at a base of 100 mg/dl and less than 140 after meals.

Note: Readers who are already using insulin will have a background of knowledge for following the next section. If you don't need multiple shots you may wish to skim this section or skip ahead. This information is easier to teach to a specific patient, building one step at a time. What follows is an explanation on learning how to use multiple injections.

WHAT IF ONE SHOT A DAY DOESN'T CONTROL MY BLOOD SUGAR LEVELS?

If your A1C level remains above 7 percent, even after you learn to lower your morning blood sugar consistently down to 100 mg/dl, it is a sign that your pancreas just can't make enough insulin on its own to respond to the pills and the single injection you are taking. This means you need more shots to mimic the normal insulin production of the pancreas.

When you start taking more than one shot of insulin you learn that you actually gain more flexibility by taking multiple injections. This can involve giving as many as four or five shots a day, which allow you to eat meals whenever you want. If you can stick to a regular schedule, where you eat the same kinds of food and exercise at the same time every day, then you can get away with fewer shots per day (usually two or three). How you make this transition is up to you and your health care team—there are many different insulin regimens. But, yet again, remember the goal is to keep your blood sugar levels as close to normal as possible.

A common progression is to go from a once-a-day-at-bedtime NPH shot to shots before breakfast and after dinner. These shots are usually a mix of slow NPH insulin plus a more rapid-acting insulin (such as regular, Humalog, or Novolog). The shorter-acting insulin balances your sugar after the meal and the NPH gives you a ten-hour base dose. If you are using regular insulin, you have to wait thirty minutes after the injection to eat. You can eat right after a shot of super-fast Humalog or Novolog.

Patients taking morning Lantus for twenty-four-hour coverage may still have high blood sugar levels after eating. These patients would add an injection of a rapid-acting insulin (Humalog or Novolog) before each meal. In this way, you can adjust your insulin dose before eating based on what you are going to eat. You aren't stuck eating the same foods at the same time of day. This type of insulin schedule is called multiple daily injections, or MDI. I have found that patients who use multiple daily injections often have better control over their blood sugars and are more content than those who do not.

THE PROS AND CONS OF INSULIN MIXTURES

Many doctors prefer premixed insulin. In premixed insulin, there are two types of insulin mixed together, usually a mix of a shorter- and a longer-acting insulin. I'm not a fan of these mixes. Through the years I've discovered that most people's lifestyles don't "fit" a premixed balance of insulin. Individuals who prefer consistent patterns of eating and doing the same things, day in, day out, may respond to a premixed insulin. But most of my patients have busy schedules and active lifestyles. They need an insulin combination that is specific to them.

I have found that most patients are quite capable of learning to mix their own insulins. Premixed insulin is easier for doctors to use; there's no need to teach their patients how to mix. And premixed insulins are useful when someone, perhaps an elderly person with vision problems, isn't able to mix his or her own insulin. But most people who are able to pay attention to their diabetes and are willing to make an effort to optimize their control usually prefer to mix insulin themselves, creating the ratios and doses that work best for any given situation.

INSULIN PUMPS IN TREATING TYPE 2 DIABETES

Insulin pumps are a unique way to treat diabetes. They are most often used by people with type 1 diabetes, but they also work for some type 2 patients. Insulin pumps are devices that attach to your body and deliver a constant supply of rapid-acting insulin through a plastic catheter. You are able to push a button and the pump can give you a larger, or "bolus," dose of insulin to cover a meal. Pumps are complicated and somewhat finicky, but they have several advantages to insulin injections. For example, if you require large doses of insulin, a pump may allow you to lower the amount of insulin you give yourself every day because less is required through the pump. Some of my patients with type 2 diabetes really love being on the pump—they feel it gives them increased flexibility with meals and exercise and, thus, helps them work on weight loss. Other people hate the idea of having something continuously attached to their body and don't want to have to do the frequent testing and troubleshooting that pumps require. If you are on frequent daily insulin injections you may want to consider an insulin pump. It's a decision that is worth discussing with your doctor. For more information on pumps, visit one of these websites: www.minimed.com, www.deltec.com, www.animas.com, www.disetronic.com.

....

"I figured that if I didn't use insulin, then I didn't have the disease."

Many of my patients eventually need to take insulin, and almost all don't want to start. What always amazes me is how expert patients become once they overcome their initial fears. Vicki really learned how to master insulin and integrate it into her life.

I was diagnosed with diabetes in 1993. Although my family on both sides (father, aunts, grandfather) had diabetes, I was convinced that I would never get it. I began to have terrible pain in my feet. In fact, it was only because the treatments I tried didn't work that I was sent to a specialist to find what the real problem was.

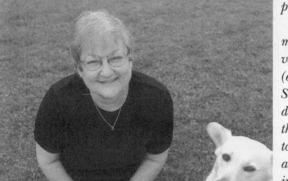

find what the real problem was.

My case didn't manifest itself in very obvious ways (except for my feet). So I spent a good deal of time ignoring the problem. I refused to go to a dietitian, and wouldn't go on insulin, even though I trusted my doctor and knew she was right to recommend injections. I figured that if I didn't use insulin, then I didn't have the disease. Once I used insulin, I reasoned, I would have to leave the safety of denial and enter the world of reality. I wasn't willing to do that—at least not then.

I credit the patience of my doctor with my turnaround. By understanding who I was and knowing not to push me, she slowly brought me around to the idea of insulin by asking me to pick a date on my own when I would be willing to try it. Since it was my decision, I picked a date about four months later. Then, as the date got closer, I got so used to the idea that I moved the date up and actually started a month early. I had no fear of needles. I just didn't want to have diabetes.

I've been on insulin for three years now. I use prefilled pens that you just shake, dial a dosage, and inject with tiny needles. It takes about two minutes of my time once a day. It's easy, and the difference in my blood sugar readings are amazing. I don't do everything I'm supposed to do to be a perfect diabetes patient. But I never get judged by anyone, so I feel as if I have the freedom to accept the disease in my own way. Because of that, I try more than if someone was forcing it on me. I'm lucky to have a great support team in my doctors, my family, and my friends. That makes a huge difference to me.

I am a very active person. My diabetes doesn't interfere with my life. I am the chair of Friends of the Culver City Dog Park, a nonprofit organization working to bring an off-leash dog park to my city. We started with six members and now have more than two thousand supporters, plus we have in excess of $44,000 in the bank—all since August 2001. Walking my dogs has been great for my diabetes, and more important, they are wonderful companions. I can't wait for them to enjoy our dog park.

....

Many people live in a state of denial of the symptoms or diagnosis of diabetes. Vicki was able to overcome this and, from her story, you can see that once she accepted the fact of diabetes her life improved. But not everyone comes around to acceptance on their own. Sadly, if left untreated, or if the wrong course of treatment is followed for too long, or even if the right course of treatment is given but not followed, the disease will make its presence felt in drastic ways. This is where the diabetes horror stories come from, the ones you've heard—and I've seen—too often. But they're not really horror stories, they are *tragedies* because *diabetic complications can be prevented.*

THIRTEEN

PREVENTING AND TREATING TYPE 2 COMPLICATIONS

Every patient I have lives in fear of the complications of diabetes. But almost all of the complications of diabetes are preventable *if* you take good care of yourself. The complications of type 2 and type 1 diabetes are the same, because the root cause is increased amounts of sugar in the bloodstream. This chapter, explaining many of the complications that can occur as a result of diabetes, may seem overwhelmingly frightening and discouraging. It's not meant to be. I think of it more as motivational because the most important thing to take from this chapter is that none of what is described *has* to occur. I want you to come away telling yourself, "This doesn't have to happen to me." Repeat: "I *can* and *will* prevent these complications from happening to my body." And even if you have early complications, in many cases, we can prevent them from becoming worse. What you need to do is to understand the risks, learn what needs to be tested and how often, and take the steps you need to take to live well with your diabetes.

On a personal note, I think that part of my passion in treating diabetes comes from the fact that I've seen all of the complications I talk about below and then some. I have firsthand experience with the worst. In fact, I deal with these conditions every day. So I am a zealot for prevention—I hate seeing people suffer. Now that we have the tools—the pills, insulins, and monitoring devices—that can allow you to lead a long and complication-free life with diabetes, there's no reason you shouldn't.

COMPLICATIONS: CAUSES AND EFFECTS

The classic complications of diabetes happen because certain parts of the body are more sensitive than others to the harmful effects of high blood sugar levels. It usually takes ten to fifteen years of having high blood sugar levels for complications to develop. But many people with type 2 diabetes have lived with high blood sugar levels for seven to ten years before the diagnosis has been made. So I regularly see patients with what is considered "newly diagnosed" diabetes who already have complications. This is reason enough in itself to be sure you are tested early and often if you are at risk for diabetes. People at risk should be sure that family members are tested for diabetes, too. I have a number of multigenerational families in my practice. I treat the complications of the grandparents, help the parents to avoid complications, and work with the grandchildren to prevent diabetes.

---

*People at risk should be sure that family members
are tested for diabetes, too.*

Diabetic complications are divided into two groups. The first group is called microvascular complications. These complications of the small blood vessels damage the eyes, kidneys, and nerves. The second group is called macrovascular (large blood vessel) complications. Such complications involve the heart and the major blood vessels throughout the body. Heart attack, stroke, and peripheral vascular disease are the potential results of these complications.

One of the areas of your body most vulnerable to microvascular complications is the retina in the back of your eyes (more on that in a moment). Diabetes also can cause significant damage to the kidneys. Diabetes is currently the number one reason people have kidney failure in the United States and the most common reason people need to go on dialysis (use an artificial kidney machine). Your entire nervous system, but most commonly the nerves in your legs and feet, can be damaged as well by high blood sugar levels. It is common for patients to complain of burning pain in their toes that gives way to numbness. This numbness in turn makes them less sensitive to pain in their feet, which can lead to ulcers (non-healing sores) on the bottoms of the feet and toes. Such ulcers have the potential to develop into an infection in the bone and can require amputation. To prevent these microvascular complications you need to lower your blood sugar levels to as close to normal as possible and keep them in that normal range. However, if these microvascular complications have already begun, there are approaches that can be taken to help slow them down.

The macrovascular complications are primarily related to abnormal lipid (cholesterol and triglyceride) levels and high blood pressure. These abnormalities, especially common in people with type 2 diabetes, can cause heart attacks, strokes, and clogging of the arteries in the legs. High blood sugar levels probably make the abnormal cholesterol and triglyceride levels more deadly. Lowering the risk of heart disease in people with diabetes, then, means targeting high blood sugar, blood pressure, and cholesterol and triglyceride levels.

TABLE 14

Body Area at Risk	Outcome If Complication Isn't Caught Early and/or Treated	How to Avoid a Serious Problem Developing	What to Do If There Are Signs of Damage
Eyes	Impairment of vision; blindness	Go at least once a year to an eye doctor who specializes in diabetes to have a *dilated* eye exam; keep blood pressure less than 130/80 mmHg.	Laser treatment; certain types of eye surgery; improve control of blood pressure.

Kidneys	Kidney failure, dialysis, kidney transplant	Every year have a urine test for microalbumin-uria. Have blood pressure tested at every doctor visit.	Use drugs such as ACE inhibitors or angiotensin receptor blockers (ARBs); maintain blood pressure at less than 130/80 mmHg; avoid drugs and treatments that can damage kidneys further.
Nerves	Severe pain syndromes; loss of a foot or leg; impotence; disorders of the bladder, stomach, and intestines	Have doctor check for damage to feet at every visit; check feet at home every day.	Once nerve damage occurs it is hard to treat, except by checking feet every day and taking pain medications
Heart	Heart attack, congestive heart failure, sudden death	Have choles-terol and triglyceride levels tested every year and treated if abnormal. Have an annual physical and a routine treadmill test.	Take a cholesterol-lowering drug, a beta-blocking drug, and an aspirin every day; make sure blood pressure is less than 130/80 mmHg.

MICROVASCULAR COMPLICATIONS: EYES (RETINOPATHY), KIDNEYS (NEPHROPATHY), AND NERVES (NEUROPATHY)

Diabetic Eye Damage

Damaged Retina

Diabetic eye disease (retinopathy) means damage to the retina, which is the inner lining of the back of the eye. The retina is a delicate, amazing nerve layer that collects the images that come through the eye's lens and sends them through specialized nerves cells to the back of your brain, where they are interpreted in the form of vision. Most people go to an optometrist because they are near- or far-sighted. The glasses or contact lenses we wear correct any difficulty in focusing images on the retina. This problem relating to the front of the eye is different from the actual damage to the back of the eye that can occur with diabetes.

Early stages of retinal damage are difficult to detect unless a professional looks in your eye all the way to the back. Often, people notice no changes in vision until the damage has advanced to involve the center of your vision. When I ask people if they have gone to the eye doctor and they tell me, "I don't have any problems seeing" or "I was just fitted for glasses so I don't need to go again," I know they don't understand the importance of a thorough retinal exam. So I use the opportunity to teach them about the silent nature of diabetic eye damage and how important it is to have an annual dilated exam performed by a different type of eye doctor, an ophthalmologist.

When you have high blood sugars for a long time, the blood vessels in the retina become fragile and break. First they rupture in just a few little spots, called "dot and blot hemorrhages." The resulting "mild background retinopathy" doesn't cause loss of vision. If blood sugar levels stay high, however, additional damage occurs and more tiny blood vessels break and bleed. Your retina can begin to swell as a reaction to the damage. If this happens at your macula, which is the center of your sight process, you can go blind in that eye. Fortunately, if your eye doctor finds that you are having problems near your macula, he or she can give you virtually painless laser therapy and stop the problem before it can cause blindness.

It has always seemed odd to me that burning the back of the eye with a laser beam can help reduce the swelling and help treat diabetic eye damage, but it does. It basically stops the blood from flowing through the damaged blood vessels and encourages normal, healthy blood flow through other capillaries at the back of the eye.

People with diabetes need to go for a dilated eye exam every year.

In some people with diabetes, the eye forms new blood vessels in an attempt to get oxygen to the back of the eye. These new blood vessels are weak and fragile and can easily break. This is called proliferative retinopathy. Leakage from these breaks fills the vitreous (gelatin) portion of the eye with blood. If this happens, sudden loss of vision can occur in the affected eye. There is not much that can be done at this point, except to wait for the blood to flush and then perform laser treatment. Sometimes surgery is needed if the eye doesn't clear. If you have a sudden loss of vision, go immediately to a retinal specialist for an evaluation.

If you have diabetes long enough, even with good control, you will probably have a few spots of retinopathy on the back of your eye. But if this damage is not in the center of your eye and is considered mild background retinopathy, it shouldn't cause you any problems. People with diabetes need to go for a dilated eye exam every year. At this exam, eyedrops are used to widen your pupils enough for the ophthalmologist to examine the back of your eye thoroughly. Most retinal specialists will keep photographic records of your eyes for future comparison to detect any changes. Just having your regular doctor look into your eyes isn't good enough—he or she could miss important developments. I look at the back of all my patients' eyes when I first meet them. I figure that if I can see any bleeding, abnormal spots, or blood vessels then serious problems could be present. I send the patient to the eye doctor right away. But even if I see nothing, I always recommend every patient see an eye doctor once a year who specializes in diabetes. Early detection and treatment is critical.

Blurry Vision When Diabetes Is First Diagnosed

When patients first get diabetes and have very high blood sugar levels, they often tell me their vision is blurry. They are understandably afraid this means that they have eye damage. The good news is that this usually isn't a serious problem at all. High blood sugar levels adversely affect the lens of the eye. The lens has the same balance of water composition as the rest of your body. When blood sugar levels go up, sugar goes everywhere, including to the lens. But sugar molecules go in and out of the lens more slowly than the rest of the body. When blood sugar levels fall in the rest of your body, the sugar level in your lens remains higher. This causes the shape of the lens to change, which distorts or alters vision. Until the blood sugar and water levels in the lens catch up to the rest of your body, vision will be a little off. It can take as long as a month for the process to stabilize. So I tell newly diagnosed people to wait before they get new glasses until they have had normal, or stable, blood sugar levels for a month. In the meantime, you can go to the store and check out the cheap, premade reading glasses to see if they help. As with all my patients, I also recommend an exam by a retinal specialist to make certain it is the front—and not the back—of the eye that is affected.

Cataracts

People with diabetes probably develop cataracts more often and at a younger age than those without diabetes. Cataracts are a clouding of the lens in the front of the eye, which can impair vision. Cataracts in people with diabetes are treated the same way everyone else's are. New surgical techniques make cataract removal safer and less invasive than ever before. People with diabetes having cataract surgery, however, should have a thorough retinal exam first. Cataract surgery can sometimes worsen diabetic eye disease so it's best to confirm that you don't have active retinopathy prior to any cataract procedure.

Diabetic Kidney Disease

High blood sugar levels and high blood pressure levels cause damage to the kidneys. If both are kept under control, your kidneys should be fine. In fact, I expect that most people I treat will never have any kidney damage. However, it is prudent to be aware of what *can* damage your kidneys and how to lower that risk.

A normal kidney is in charge of filtering blood and making urine. It keeps the salts and water in the body in balance. And it makes hormones that circulate throughout the body and regulate blood pressure. It also makes erythropoietin, which helps regulate the number of red blood cells in the body. Those are big responsibilities. Most of us are born with two functioning kidneys, although some people are born with only one. It doesn't matter if you have one or two because, as kidney donors illustrate, one can handle all that needs to be done.

I expect that most people I treat will never have any kidney damage.

Under a microscope a kidney is a beautiful organ, filled with ducts and swirls of cells that work to filter the blood. When high blood sugar damages the kidneys, it starts to kill some of these cells needed for normal function. The kidneys then start to leak albumin, or protein, into your urine, which signals they are impaired and are no longer able to effectively filter blood and urine. One of the first ways we can detect kidney damage is to measure the leakage of albumin into a urine sample.

If you have early untreated kidney damage, the slight loss of albumin in the urine starts to increase. The affected kidney first becomes more and more like a sieve and then loses all ability to filter your blood. This causes your blood pressure to rise and the creatinine level in your blood to increase. This is the last measure of kidney dysfunction. Once your creatinine level rises above normal, your kidneys have been permanently damaged and are not working at a normal rate. However, even at this stage you can make a positive impact on your kidney function. With blood pressure treatment, medications, and meticulous control of blood sugar you can stabilize your kidneys, or at least slow down the rate at which they deteriorate. The goal is to keep your kidneys working well enough to filter your blood without the necessity of dialysis.

If your kidneys keep getting worse and worse and your creatinine level rises to 3 or 4 mg/dl (anything below 1.4–1.5 is considered normal), you will be nearing the required level for dialysis. In dialysis you are attached on a regular schedule to a machine that works as a filter for your blood. Dialysis can be difficult, but it does work. Another option is to have a kidney transplant, as a number of my patients have done. Obviously, you never want to end up on dialysis, or to be on a wait list for a transplant, or to have to ask a relative or friend to be a kidney donor. Open and honest discussions are encouraged with your physician about your kidney function and what to expect if problems are developing.

The Kidney–Blood Pressure Connection

There is a direct relationship between kidney damage and blood pressure. So for kidney health, you not only need to keep your blood sugar levels normal, you need to keep your blood pressure level under control, as well. When the kidneys become damaged blood pressure goes up, and this increase in blood pressure further damages your kidneys. This is one of the reasons the standards for blood pressure in people with diabetes are stricter than for people without diabetes. I start treatment if blood pressure is more than 130/80 mmHg and try to keep your blood pressure well below that level. (People without diabetes are allowed to have a level below 140/90 mmHg.) Along with its association with kidney damage and retinopathy, high blood pressure—in people with and without diabetes—increases the risk for macrovascular complications: heart damage, heart attack, and stroke. Have your blood pressure checked at every office visit. There's a good reason why it is so routinely done.

Once a year, you should have a urine test and a blood test done to be sure your kidneys show no signs of damage. Or, if there already is damage, you need to make sure it isn't getting worse. The test for your urine is called an albumin to creatinine (A/C) ratio, or a microalbumin (MA) test. We used to make every patient collect their urine for twenty-four hours so we could measure how much protein leaked out. Now we can do it in a single sample you give at the doctor's office. Sometimes a twenty-four-hour urine collection is needed, but less often than in the past.

There are many different names for this A/C ratio or MA test and not enough doctors who perform it. Fewer than one in ten of my patients who come from other doctors with their lab reports have had this test done. The more common test doctors do is called a urine test for protein. This test tells you whether or not you have very serious kidney damage. But at the point this urine test shows positive for protein, you probably have had kidney damage for several years. Because the standard tests don't pick up early damage, it is important to have the test done for microalbuminuria, which does.

If the albumin to creatinine ratio is greater than 30, it may be a sign that there is some early damage to your kidneys. I strongly suggest you have it measured twice, to confirm that you really have a problem. Note that there can be false positive results if you have an infection in your bladder or urine, which can make it look like you have protein in your urine when you don't. Or if you have blood in your urine (if you are a female having your period) the test also can show a false leakage of protein. With either condition present, you may want to wait until your next doctor visit so you can give a clean urine sample. If your urine tests for microalbumin or protein are positive, you should start taking an angiotensin-converting enzyme inhibitor (ACE inhibitor) and/or angiotensin receptor blocker (ARB). Both drugs were made for treating high blood pressure but have been shown to have the additional benefit of slowing the rate of kidney failure in people with diabetes—whether the existing damage is early (microalbuminuria) or late (proteinuria). These drugs are helpful whether or not an increase of blood pressure is present. However, be aware that if your blood pressure is usually low your health care provider should start you on only a very low dose of these medications to avoid having them cause your blood pressure to fall *too* low.

The ACE inhibitors tend to work quite well, and are available as lower-cost generic agents, but may cause a dry cough that can be quite annoying. If this happens you can be switched to an ARB, which doesn't have this effect. Keep in mind, however, if you have a cough from an ACE inhibitor it can take a month for it to go away. Sometimes when people are switched from an ACE inhibitor to an ARB and the cough doesn't immediately go away, they think the ARB is causing a cough as well. That isn't true—it's just that the ACE inhibitor cough hasn't gone away yet.

If you have a cough from an ACE inhibitor it can take a month for it to go away.

A side effect common to both ACE inhibitors and ARBs is an increase in blood potassium levels. Normal potassium level is usually around 4 mEq/L. These drugs often increase the potassium level in people with diabetes to 5 mEq/L or greater. A potassium level of 6 mEq/L can be deadly, so be sure your potassium level is checked a month or so after being started on an ACE inhibitor or an ARB and then followed, particularly if it is increasing. High potassium levels can be treated, but do need to be detected.

The use of ACE inhibitors and ARBs is not always adequate to bring blood pressure into the normal range of 130/80 mmHg or less. It often takes three or more medications to control blood pressure in patients with diabetes. Patients are generally started on an ACE inhibitor or an ARB. Then a diuretic such as hydrochlorothiazide (HCTZ) is added. If that doesn't work, other classes of medications, most commonly beta-blockers or calcium channel blockers, are prescribed. Usually if I can't control blood pressure easily with three medications, or if a patient's creatinine level is above 2 mg/dl, I have the patient see a kidney specialist (a nephrologist). I work with some excellent kidney specialists, and together we can often keep a patient's kidneys functioning for many years.

Commonly Used ACE Inhibitors

Generic Name	Brand Names
benazepril	Lotensin
captopril	Capoten

enalapril	Vasotec
fosinopril	Monopril
lisinopril	Prinivil, Zestril
moexipril	Univasc
perinodopril	Aceon
quinapril	Accupril
ramipril	Altace
trandolapril	Mavik

Commonly Used ARBs

Generic Name	Brand Names
candesartan	Atacand, Atacand HCT*
eprosartan	Teveten, Teveten HCT*
irbesartan	Avapro, Avalide*
losartan	Cozaar, Hyzaar*
olmesartan	Benicar, Benicar HCT*
tasosartan	Verdia
telmisartan	Micardis, Micardis HCT*
valsartan	Diovan, Diovan HCT*

Diabetic Nerve Damage

Of all the diabetes complications I treat, nerve damage may be the most distressing. Neuropathy, like all of the complications, has many different stages. Fewer treatment options, however, are available at each stage. The best strategy of all is to prevent nerve damage

---

*Hydrochlorothiazide added to ARB

by keeping blood sugar levels normal. But if neuropathy does develop it is important to understand what it is, what to expect, and what can be done to help.

The list of all the types of neuropathy caused by diabetes is very long. Basically diabetes can affect any of the nerves in your body. Some nerves are more vulnerable to damage from diabetes than others. I will focus on the main groups, but it is possible to have other nerves involved.

Knowing what nerves do makes understanding diabetic neuropathy easier. Nerves carry signals to and from all parts of your body to create a feedback loop that allows your brain to know what is happening and control the body. Your brain and spinal cord make up the central nervous system—the main system for relaying and processing nerve signals. You also have a peripheral nervous system that includes the nerve fibers running down your legs and arms. And, last, you have what is called an autonomic nervous system, which sends signals to keep your internal organs working, such as your stomach, intestines, and heart. Much of our nervous system is on autopilot, constantly sending signals back through the central nervous system to help coordinate our actions.

Nerve Damage to the Feet

One important function of nerves is to tell us that we are injured. Pain is a signal that something is wrong, as well as a call to action. When nerves become damaged by diabetes, the lining of the nerves starts to die. This causes the nerves to register pain. This type of painful nerve damage starts in the toes and feet and is called peripheral sensory polyneuropathy. Basically, what it means is that the longest and most vulnerable nerves in your body, the nerves to your toes and feet, are losing function. The next nerves that most commonly are damaged are the ones that extend to the fingertips. Another name for this type of nerve damage is "stocking-glove" neuropathy.

The pain of this type of neuropathy is often worse at night. Patients who have it can't sleep because the pain, often a burning sensation, is so severe. High blood sugar levels seem to worsen the pain. Lowering blood sugar levels may help lessen the pain, although it cannot repair the damage. The pain of neuropathy generally requires additional treatment. One of the most effective medications to treat this pain is gabapentin (Neurontin), which helps calm the irritation of the nerves. Other medications can also be used, such as drugs used to treat depression (like Elavil, desipramine, Prozac, Effexor, and Cymbalta) and drugs used to treat seizures (Tegretol and Topamax). Over time, the pain will dissipate, but that can take years. And when the pain is gone it means the nerves have died and are no longer sending signals to your brain. Your feet end up feeling numb, making you more susceptible to ulcers and infections of the bone. In the worst case this can lead to amputation. Once your feet are painful or numb the nerve damage can't be reversed. Prevention is crucial.

Numbness is tested by your doctor with a touch to the bottom of your foot with something called a monofilament. If you can't feel this as a sort of light tickling, you can't feel pokes and cuts to your feet. This means that your eyes have to become your nerves and you must check the bottoms of your feet twice a day to be sure there are no new cuts or sores that need attention from a member of your health care team.

Nerve Damage to the Intestines, Stomach, and Bladder

Although most people don't realize it, the most common symptom of diabetic nerve damage may be constipation, caused by damage to the nerves that go to the intestines. Damage to the intestinal nerves also can cause diarrhea as well as a buildup of bacteria in the gut. Another troubling problem can involve the nerves of the stomach. If these nerves are damaged, the stomach doesn't empty normally and food can build up, causing gastroparesis, a feeling of bloating and nausea, and sometimes vomiting. As you can imagine, this makes management of diabetes more difficult because food is absorbed unpredictably—often too slowly—and judging insulin doses becomes difficult. Persistent gastroparesis may be helped by giving rapid-acting insulin after, instead of before, meals.

There are some medications useful in treating gastroparesis; change of diet also can help. High blood sugar levels, the source of the problem in the first place, may intensify gastroparesis. As always, good control can make a big difference. I also recommend seeing a gastroenterologist if you have this problem so you can receive the most up-to-date treatment available.

The nerves to the bladder also are liable to be damaged by diabetes. If this happens, your bladder may not empty normally, causing urine to build up. Frequent bladder infections can result, which can be treated with antibiotics and certain medications that can improve the bladder's ability to function.

Erectile Dysfunction

Part of the questionnaire I have new patients fill out asks whether or not they have problems with sexual function. All too often male patients have checked the "yes" box. But it can take several visits before a new patient feels comfortable enough to talk with me about the problem. What most people don't realize is that I talk about sexual dysfunction with my patients all the time. There is very little I haven't heard and often I can help. Yet I know how sensitive an issue it is, and understand if a patient is hesitant to bring it up. Sexual performance problems are difficult for men to discuss with anyone—let alone a doctor who is a woman.

Erectile dysfunction (ED) affects up to half of all men who have diabetes. This is due to nerve damage, as well as damage to the blood vessels that go to the penis. This complication is exceptionally unfortunate because it is completely preventable by good control of blood sugar levels, cholesterol, and blood pressure. You've probably heard of drugs such as Viagra, Levitra, and Cialis (it's difficult to avoid commercials for them). Though the action of each has distinguishing characteristics, they all work basically the same way—to dilate blood vessels and increase blood flow to the penis. All can aid or improve sexual function and won't negatively affect your diabetes. Improving your blood sugar levels also can help, even if there has been some prior damage.

Sexual performance problems are difficult for men to discuss with anyone—let alone a doctor who is a woman.

Less Common Symptoms of Neuropathy

The types of neuropathy mentioned above are all due to damage caused by chronic increases in blood sugar levels over time. (We believe that the nerves are gradually damaged and that once the damage happens it can't be reversed.) Another type of neuropathy happens when a blood vessel to a nerve suddenly becomes clogged. The process isn't clear yet, but sometimes just that one nerve turns off. Function in that affected nerve does return, usually after six to twelve months.

I had a sweet young man in his mid twenties come to see me for diabetes care, who had never been willing to see a diabetes specialist before. He was motivated to come because he lost the ability to move his right eye from side to side. He worked as a cameraman, and was particularly worried about the double vision his neuropathy was causing. I was able to reassure him that his vision would become normal over time, and within six months he was as good as new. Meanwhile, I tried to convince him to take better care of his diabetes control. This didn't happen immediately, but a year later he broke his elbow when some camera boxes fell. While recovering from the injury he had lots of time to monitor his blood sugar levels, learn diabetes management, and improve his diabetes control. You never know what the trigger will be to get you to pay attention to your diabetes, but it is always better to get good control sooner rather than later.

MACROVASCULAR COMPLICATIONS: HEART DISEASE, VASCULAR DISEASE, HIGH BLOOD PRESSURE, AND STROKE

While the microvascular complications of diabetes cause much suffering and disability, it is the macrovascular complications that can kill you. Up to 80 percent of people with diabetes will die from diseases of the heart and blood vessels. Unlike the eye, kidney, and nerve damage that is directly caused by high blood sugar levels that you can change, other, less readily controlled, factors are involved in complications of the heart and blood vessels. Macrovascular complications are caused by a complex interaction of high blood sugar level, abnormal cholesterol and triglyceride levels, and high blood pressure. Modifiable risk factors, including cigarette smoking, obesity, and inactivity, raise the risk for heart disease in people with diabetes just as they impact people without diabetes.

Up to 80 percent of people with diabetes will die from diseases of the heart and blood vessels.

The risk of heart disease in patients with type 2 diabetes is so high—at least double that of someone without diabetes—that almost all of them need medication to reduce the probability of heart disease. For instance, a patient may boast of a cholesterol level of 200 mg/dl. But in my head I'm doubling that number to 400. That's the way the numbers work for people with diabetes. And almost everyone will concede that a cholesterol reading of 400 is too high.

As with the microvascular complications of diabetes, prevention of macrovascular complications is preferred over treatment. Before discussing the use of medication to prevent macrovascular disease in people with diabetes, you must understand the overall problems and risks.

There are four main types of macrovascular disease: heart disease, stroke, high blood pressure, and peripheral vascular disease. The heart disease I'm most concerned with is called coronary artery disease (CAD), or clogging of the arteries that supply blood to the heart. A slow clogging of these blood vessels can cause symptoms such as angina (chest pain brought on by activity or exercise) or sudden interruption of the blood supply to the heart, causing pain and the death of part of the heart muscle. In the worst-case scenario, the person with CAD suddenly dies because the heart's rhythm has been so badly disturbed.

Short of death, a clogged artery can cause a heart attack, which can lead to permanent damage to your heart. There are treatments that can save your life and your heart if you get to an emergency room IMMEDIATELY upon having symptoms of a heart attack; the clot that caused the attack must be quickly dissolved before the heart muscle dies. Symptoms of a heart attack include a feeling of pain or pressure in the left side of your chest, often accompanied by pain radiating into your left arm or jaw. Sometimes you feel shortness of breath, sweating, and nausea along with the pain, but sometimes you can have no pain and just shortness of breath and nausea by itself. If you have these symptoms go to an emergency room immediately for treatment.

You want to be aware of any macrovascular complications long before you have a heart attack. You should have regular treadmill tests to see if the blood vessels to your heart are open and providing enough blood for your heart to function normally. If there is any problem, you will have a cardiac catheterization. In this procedure the doctor (a cardiologist, or heart specialist) feeds thin plastic tubing (a catheter) into a major blood vessel in your groin (near the junction of your upper leg and pelvis). The catheter is guided into your heart and through it dye is injected. This dye runs through the arteries in your heart and shows if there are any narrowings or clogs. If the narrowings are severe your doctor will try to open them. Some clogs are opened by simply squeezing through the narrowing and then expanding the area with a balloon placed on the end of catheter (a procedure called angioplasty). Other clogs are treated by inserting a "stent" (a little cylindrical device that looks like a small coil). Sometimes this stent has been coated with antibiotics or an anti-inflammatory drug. In general, stenting is better than just angioplasty in patients with diabetes, because people with diabetes have a higher than normal rate of artery closing after the procedure, but you need to trust your cardiologist to make these decisions for you.

You should have regular treadmill tests to see if the blood vessels to your heart are open and providing enough blood for your heart to function normally.

If angioplasty or stenting doesn't work, or your arteries are severely plugged, you will be sent for coronary bypass grafting, or CABG bypass surgery. In this procedure a vein is taken from your leg or arm (or the arteries inside your chest are used) and blood flow is rerouted around the clogged arteries. Depending on your condition, the surgeons may need to bypass one, two, three, or more of the vessels in your heart. Obviously, this is a major operation, although it is increasingly common, and you will want the best cardiac surgeon you can find to perform it. Different hospitals have different rates of success. Find a surgeon who does these procedures very often—at least several times per week, and can tell you his or her outcomes. Ask how many CABGs he or she does per year, how many patients die, and how many patients have serious problems after surgery. Often there are surgeons that everyone knows— I can think of several in Los Angeles who are really great. You need to ask your cardiologist and your internist for their recommendations. Ask why they like the surgeon they are choosing. Often going to a university medical center where experts work is a good place for such an involved procedure. Careful research is necessary.

Treatments to Lower the Risk for Heart Disease in People with Diabetes

Here is the bottom line.

If you have type 2 diabetes you should take:

1. A statin

2. An aspirin

3. An ACE inhibitor or ARB

These three classes of drugs are so helpful (actually they're beyond helpful—they're life-saving), most patients with diabetes should be taking them in addition to medications to lower blood sugar levels. Some people also benefit from a fibric acid derivative or a niacin supplement to lower their triglycerides.

Statins to Lower Cholesterol

There have been many studies of the benefits of cholesterol-lowering drugs called statins (such as Mevacor, Lescol, Pravachol, Zocor, Lipitor, Crestor). I think I can speak for the majority of my fellow physicians when I say, the more we use these drugs the more we like them. At first, these drugs were administered to only those people who had very high cholesterol levels. When the statins helped these people, the indications for treatment using them were lowered. Statins have been shown to lower the risk of heart disease at all cholesterol levels in people with diabetes and can reduce the risk for heart attack by about 30 percent. The Heart Protection Study (HPS) found that giving a statin to people with diabetes (in this case Zocor) lowered the risk of heart attack no matter what the level of cholesterol. The CARDS study showed that a low dose of Lipitor given to patients with diabetes also lowered the risk of heart attack, even in patients with a low baseline cholesterol level.

The risk for heart attack and stroke is so high I feel strongly that everyone with type 2 diabetes should be on a statin. Bringing LDL (bad) cholesterol level to less than 100 mg/dl is ideal. Aiming for an LDL of 60 to 70 is even better, especially for anyone who's recently had a heart attack. More and more studies are suggesting that lower is better when it comes to LDL cholesterol. We do, however, need *some* cholesterol for our bodies to function so there may be a limit (that we haven't figured out yet) that is too low to maintain safely.

Many people aren't aware that statins can cause muscle pain, and this is not something that is often picked up in a lab test, so it is important to let your doctor know if you have this when you start on a statin.

The statin drugs work to prevent the body from making excess cholesterol. Because your body is busiest making cholesterol while you are sleeping, we recommend that you take statin at bedtime. The potential side effects to the statins include damage to the liver and muscles. This sounds awful, but the benefits to your cholesterol levels (and therefore your heart) far outweigh the risks. Liver damage, if it occurs, is usually mild and can be easily picked up by a blood test. The statin should be stopped; the liver damage is not permanent. The muscle problem is more common but not life-threatening, and generally manifests itself in muscle pain and achiness not related to exercise or other illness. Many people aren't aware that statins can cause muscle pain, and this is not something that is often picked up in a lab test, so it is important to let your doctor know if you have this when you start on a statin. Sometimes switching from one type of statin to another can help diminish or eliminate the pain.

There is also another drug for lowering cholesterol, called Zetia, that is probably not as good as a statin at lowering heart attack risk, but can be used if you can't take a statin (or added to the statin) if your cholesterol doesn't come down enough. The only other side effect that I see in people using statins with any frequency is a change in their dreams. Sometimes people say their dreams are more vivid, or they have more nightmares. An occasional patient (usually with a history of depression or bipolar illness) will say that they can't take statins because the changes in their dreams are too intense or it affects their moods.

Ways to Lower Triglycerides and Raise HDL Levels

It's an established fact that lowering cholesterol is critical to any treatment hoping to reduce the risk of heart attack, stroke, and vascular disease. So what can people with type 2 diabetes do about problem LDL (bad) cholesterol, elevated triglyceride levels, and low levels of HDL (good) cholesterol?

The first steps are to lower blood sugar levels and insulin resistance by losing weight, increasing exercise, and taking medication for diabetes (particularly a drug like Actos). If you do this, plus take a statin drug to lower cholesterol level, you may not have to do anything else.

Other options involve taking a class of drugs known as fibric acid derivatives. The two drugs most commonly used are gemfibrozil (Lopid) and fenofibrate (Tricor). These drugs lower triglyceride levels and heart disease risk, although maybe not quite as much as statins do. You can take Tricor along with a statin, but this increases the risk of serious muscle and liver damage and your doctor needs to monitor you closely.

Niacin also works very well to lower triglyceride levels and increase HDL cholesterol, but may make insulin resistance worse. I use niacin more often in treating people without diabetes than with diabetes, but if your blood sugars are followed closely it is a possibility. Like anyone using niacin, you will need to start at a low dose and increase it gradually to lessen the rate of flushing that can occur. Taking an aspirin before taking the niacin can help lower the incidence of flushing. I often prescribe a long-acting niacin, such as Niaspan, because it causes less flushing.

With both fibrates and niacin you should have your liver function measured twelve weeks after starting on the drugs and then again after three months or so. Remember that almost any drug you're taking can affect your liver, so be sure to have your liver function tested at least once or twice a year.

Aspirin: Not Just for Headaches

When you have diabetes your blood is simply more likely to clot. Now consider that a heart attack or stroke commonly involves both a narrowing of the blood vessels (from cholesterol and inflammation) and a sudden clogging of the blood vessels from a clot. It's pretty easy to see, then, that anything that can safely help reduce clotting in people with diabetes is worth a look. This is exactly what aspirin does, by thinning the blood. Modern medicine still isn't sure which dose of aspirin is best; common sense dictates the higher the dose, the less the chance of clotting. But aspirin is tough on the stomach, and with higher doses there is more of a chance of causing bleeding, particularly from stomach ulcers.

I tell patients to start on a baby aspirin (81 mg) every day. Look for coated versions made for adults that are more stomach-friendly. On this minor dose there may be a slight increase in bleeding and bruising—unsettling indicators of the good effect happening inside your blood vessels—but not so much that it is distressing. I personally take a baby aspirin with calcium. I started with one every day, but on this dose I got a lot of bruising on my legs. I then decreased the frequency to taking one every Monday, Wednesday, and Friday. It is hard to remember to take something every other day, but taking it on fixed days helps. And, by the way, taking Tylenol, Advil, or any other pain reliever is not a substitute for daily aspirin; they are different compounds.

Anyone who has had a bleeding problem, especially an ulcer, or who is on a drug like Coumadin, should definitely consult their doctor before taking aspirin. If you are scheduled to have surgery, you will need to stop your aspirin two weeks before the procedure to prevent extra bleeding. This is also something you should discuss with your surgeon or primary care doctor before any other medical procedures.

ACE Inhibitors and Angiotensin Receptor Blockers (ARBs)

ACE inhibitors and ARBs, in addition to slowing the progression of kidney disease (as previously mentioned in the discussion of microvascular complications), can reduce the risk of heart attacks. In a big study called the HOPE (Heart Outcomes Protection and Events) study, an ACE inhibitor called ramipril (Altace) was used in patients with diabetes or underlying heart disease. In the patients with diabetes, ramipril reduced the risk of having a heart attack and dying. This was not because it lowers blood pressure, but rather because it causes an improvement in the lining of the blood vessels. Think of the interior of healthy blood vessels as being lined with Teflon. With the development of diabetes the once-slick interior walls become more like Velcro and collect particles causing plugs or clogs. The ACE inhibitors, and probably ARBs as well, help to transform the Velcro back into Teflon.

Because of the HOPE study and other, smaller studies with ARBs, many physicians recommend that all people with type 2 diabetes take an ACE inhibitor, or an ARB if they can't tolerate an ACE inhibitor, to reduce the risk of heart disease. The starting dose with a normal blood pressure is the lowest one possible. Taking the drug at bedtime may be a good idea, in case it causes your blood pressure to drop and you get a little bit dizzy. A month or two after you start on the medication you should have blood drawn to measure your blood creatinine level and potassium to be sure these stay normal.

Peripheral Vascular Disease

Peripheral vascular disease involves clogging of the blood vessels that spread throughout the body, most often to the legs and feet.

TABLE 15. DRUGS USED FOR LOWERING MACROVASCULAR RISK

Drug classes noted in italics are those that most, if not all, patients with type 2 diabetes should take.
Older patients with type 1 diabetes may also benefit.

Drug Effect	Drug Class	Generic Name	Trade Name	Effects	Monitoring
Lipid lowering	*Statins*	Lovastatin* Pravastatin Fluvastatin Simvastatin Atorvastatin Rosuva-statin	Mevacor Pravachol Lescol Zocof Lipitor Crestor	Lowers cholesterol and inflam-mation of blood months, vessels. Lowers risk of heart attack, stroke, and death, especially muscle in people with diabetes.	Liver tests after six weeks, three months, six months, and then at least once a year. Can cause muscle pain.
	Fibric acid derivatives	Gemfibrozil* statin	Lopid	Lowers triglyceride levels. Shown to lower risk of heart attack in select patients.	Liver tests after six weeks, three months, six months, and then at least once a year. Rarely causes muscle pain.

Drug Effect	Drug Class	Generic Name	Trade Name	Effects	Monitoring
		Fenfibrate	Tricor	Lowers triglyceride levels. Shown to lower risk of heart attack in select patients.	Liver tests after six weeks, three months, six months, and then at least once a year. Rarely causes muscle pain.
	B-vitamin	Niacin*	Niaspan	Lowers triglyceride and LDL cholesterol levels; raises HDL cholesterol levels	Liver monitoring at six weeks, three months, six months, and then at least once a year. Can increase blood sugar levels. Often causes flushing.
	Cholesterol absorption inhibitors	Ezetimide	Zetia	Lowers cholesterol	None.
Reduces risk for blood clotting		Aspirin*	Many brands	Lowers the risk of heart attack and stroke.	None, but don't take if you have a problem with ulcers or other bleeding problems.
Blood pressure lowering		ACE inhibitors* and ARBs	Many—see preceding list on page 226–227	Help improve the lining of the blood vessels. Lowers blood pressure. Reduces the risk of heart attack and death.	Measure creatinine and potassium four to six weeks after starting. ACE inhibitors can cause cough.

*Available as generics

The first sign that blood flow is compromised is the decrease or loss of the pulses in the feet. Patients may complain of pain in the calves that happens after walking a certain distance. This is called claudication, and it means that there is not enough blood flow to the calf muscles. This pain goes away with rest, and then restarts with too much exercise. Like all of the other vascular complications, peripheral vascular disease occurs more often in patients with diabetes than in those without. It can be particularly dangerous in people who have peripheral neuropathy because a loss of both sensation and blood flow to the feet greatly increases the risk for amputation.

Taking statins is particularly helpful with vascular disease. If you have vascular disease and smoke, you *must* stop because smoking adversely affects the blood vessels, again increasing amputation risk. A gentle exercise program is also useful and can help the body grow new blood vessels to the feet. If the peripheral blood flow becomes severely compromised, a vascular surgeon can put in stents or do bypass surgery to help improve blood flow.

....

"'Diet, Insulin, and Exercise' were the cornerstones of my treatment."

My inspiration as a diabetologist comes from my patients, the vast majority of whom lead long and healthy lives in spite of having diabetes. This is Robert's story. He's one of my many patients who has had diabetes for more than fifty years and is still going strong.

In March 1944, shortly after my sixteenth birthday and when I was a junior in high school, I came down with a form of the flu that led to the classic signs of diabetes (although I didn't know them at the time). I was thirsty, urinated frequently, and at various times experienced blurred vision. At the time, I was working part-time as a "stack boy" at the Smith College library. Often I would feel weak and have difficulty reading the blurred letter/number designations on the book spines. I would stop working and head for a nearby drugstore for an ice cream cone, which seemed to alleviate the weakness and the blurred vision. Always an independent person, it was my nature not to share this information with anyone until I finally discussed these annoying symptoms with my dad.

My dad immediately recognized the classic signs of diabetes and brought home some copper sulfate, a test tube, and a dropper. He mixed my urine with the blue copper sulfate solution and put it into boiling water. The five minutes we had to wait seemed like an eternity and in the end the color of the fluid had turned brick red—meaning

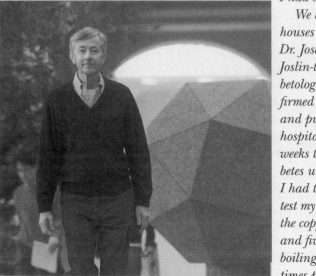

I had diabetes.

We lived several houses away from Dr. Joseph Fallon, a Joslin-trained diabetologist, who confirmed the diagnosis and put me in the hospital for two weeks to get my diabetes under control. I had to learn how to test my urine (with the copper sulfate and five minutes of boiling) four to six times per day. I learned the importance of weighing food and following the diet regimen, which would later be provided to me. I used an orange and a syringe to practice giving injections. I was taught the importance of sterilizing my glass syringe and needle in boiling water, as well as keeping the needle point sharpened.

I was given a handbook on diabetes, written by the Boston pioneer diabetologist Joslin, and in it I learned there was no permanent cure for my disease. According to the book, "Diet, Insulin, and Exercise" were the cornerstones of my treatment. I was never to forget this, and it has helped me to this day.

Not all the Joslin statements were helpful. One said, "If you are given an apple, throw it away." This seemed particularly cruel (and

*later turned out to be unnecessary) because I used to climb trees with
my friends in the fall to get McIntosh apples, which were my favorite. It
took me many years to forget their apple bias, even though I eventually
met Elliot and Allan Joslin in their Boston clinic.*

*One night, when I was lying in my hospital bed, I saw orderlies
and nurses rushing a patient into the bed across the aisle from mine.
Curtains were drawn. Then my no-nonsense diabetologist appeared
outside the curtains, walked over to my bed, and said, "See that older
patient over there? He's an insulin-taking diabetic, just like you. You
know why he's been rushed here? Because he is in a diabetic coma. He
works in a candy store and eats candy all the time and doesn't watch
his diet. He could die. Learn from this, young man." And I did. For a
lifetime.*

*It is now sixty years later. I have had a good life. I married and
raised a family and worked at the Jet Propulsion Laboratories in
Pasadena, California. I have gone from using copper sulfate to test my
urine, to using urine dipsticks (which were very inaccurate) to the
much more accurate method of measuring fingerstick blood sugar levels.
I have progressed through the types of insulin, until thanks to the new
Lantus and Humalog I have the best control of my life. And never
have I forgotten "Diet, Insulin, and Exercise." I have lived sixty
diabetic years by embracing those three words, with a lot of emphasis
on exercise. At seventy-six years old, I walk four miles a day and have
no complications of my diabetes. My only medications are insulin and
a baby aspirin that I take every day. Now I am looking forward to my
next seventy-six years!*

....

Robert is an inspiration. And there's no reason you can't be just
like him—healthy and free from complications many years after
you are diagnosed with diabetes. When he was diagnosed with diabetes, treatment was much harder and more restrictive than it is
now. Within a few years we will have even better tools for treating
diabetes and preventing complications.

Although I'd love to see diabetes cured in our lifetime, I don't
know that that will happen. What I do know is that we already have
the tools to prevent many of the complications diabetes can cause.

You are in charge of your health; you can follow your markers for complications to be sure you obtain early treatment at the first sign of any damage. Know what the complications are, how to test for them, and how to treat them. Early and aggressive detection is the best medicine, second only to prevention.

Those are doctor's orders.

PART FOUR

MASTERING TYPE 1 DIABETES

FOURTEEN

TYPE 1: THE *OTHER* DIABETES

Type 1 diabetes is basically a simple disease: your body ceases to make insulin so the insulin you need must be replaced by means of insulin injections. If you have type 1 diabetes you are completely dependent on insulin for life (or until we find a cure). This is different from the situation of people with type 2 diabetes. Type 2 individuals have both insulin resistance and insulin deficiency, and some may need insulin shots, but pills, weight loss, and exercise play the biggest roles in type 2 diabetes treatment.

Though type 1 diabetes is much less common than type 2 diabetes, it often has a more dramatic start. The classic example of someone who gets type 1 diabetes is a skinny kid who over the course of a month or so becomes very ill, loses weight, and has an increasing, insatiable thirst. Usually, there is no family history of diabetes, so the child's parents don't know to watch out for it. By the time the child is brought to the doctor or the emergency room the child is very sick, usually with a condition known as diabetic ketoacidosis (DKA). DKA happens when there is so little insulin in the body that the body breaks down fat for fuel. Too much fat breakdown leads to the excessive buildup of acids in the blood called ketones, which can cause serious problems if not treated.

For the person with diabetes and his or her family the diagnosis of diabetes can come as a complete and devastating shock. Suddenly their lives turn into a crash course on diabetes. All of the information about what to eat, what high and low blood sugar levels mean, how to test blood sugars, and how to give insulin injections must be assimilated over the course of a week. Usually this week is spent in the hospital, teaching the patient about the basics of diabetes and how to manage it once they are sent home. This is a lot to deal with all at once—especially if the patient is a child. Everyone in the family needs lots of help and support as they learn to cope with the sudden diagnosis and what it will mean for their lives going forward. Jim Natal's story is classic for an adult patient diagnosed with type 1 diabetes—generally symptoms exist for months before the diagnosis is made and once diabetes is diagnosed blood sugar levels are quite high. He found some relief from the shock of diagnosis by writing poetry. Now a successful poet who has published several books, Jim has formed a grudging truce with his diabetes, dealing with it every day as he must and dreaming of the day when it is cured.

....

"The diagnosis of diabetes tore my life apart."

I was thirty in 1978, when I was diagnosed with type 1 diabetes. I was at a low point in my life—floundering as a writer and on unemployment, which strained my already troubled marriage. I had suspected something was medically out of kilter for years because of what I now know were prediabetic hypoglycemic reactions. But I was always athletic, and at the time was playing a lot of tennis and running, which probably kept me fitter (physically and mentally) than I would otherwise have been. Then I suddenly began to drop weight. I could eat anything and not put on any pounds! In my generally overweight family this just didn't happen. After the novelty of unlimited cookies and ice cream wore off, I knew something was wrong, a suspicion that was magnified when I realized I had lost 35 pounds, was drinking liquids by the quart, and had started getting up every night to pee every couple of hours.

I had a great GP at the time who tested me and sent me to a top practice of diabetes specialists. They wasted no time in putting me on insulin; a few minutes after walking in the door I was practicing injections. I will never forget the kindness of the nurse educator I worked with. To this day, I think of her as an angel (really). But the diagnosis of diabetes tore my life apart. It was a tough time, one that it took me many years to deal with in my poetry. But, looking back, that diagnosis marked a new beginning for me in so many ways—I'm remarried,

*have a wonderful daughter, worked for twenty-five years in a dream
job as a creative executive for the NFL, and have published two, going
on three, poetry collections. And, with Dr. Peters' guidance, aggressive
and enlightened treatment approach, and prodding, I am healthier
than I would be without diabetes.*

Learning to Live with It

*Barbara taught me to give injections
to an orange, thick pop of penetration
through the skin, short smooth glide
into soft tissue under. Slowly, with control,
push down on the plunger, and quick
backward dart toss, remove the syringe.*

*I practiced in her office, still dazed from
diagnosis, seeing through pinpoint pupils,
eyes after a strobe flash. Stretched like surgical
tubing colorless with tension, I was renamed
after a disease, days now measured in gleaming
needle pricks, insulin units, blood sugar levels.*

*My wife sobbed in the car parked beneath
the medical building, rusty pipes wrapped and
painted white, strung along the oppressive ceiling.
She cried because we didn't have much money.
For the money, not for me. In that time of change
there were changes yet to come.*

*Barbara said I would learn to manage it by myself.
She said I had no choice.*

WHEN BETA CELLS DIE: THE CAUSE OF TYPE 1 DIABETES

In type 1 diabetes the cells in your pancreas responsible for se-
creting insulin, the beta cells, are destroyed. This usually does not
mean that your whole pancreas is gone (unless you have had it

surgically removed). Your pancreas is an organ that is located in the middle of your body, just behind your stomach, nestled in the crook of your small intestine as it leaves the stomach. It looks slightly like a large tadpole or a comma, with a head and a tail. Most of the pancreas's job is to secrete enzymes (special substances that break down food) into your intestines when you eat. These enzymes help digest your food. If your pancreas is removed or damaged by a disease like cystic fibrosis, you have to take enzyme pills every time you eat so you can digest your food.

In type 1 diabetes, the body gets confused and makes a major mistake.

Scattered in the tissue that makes the digestive enzymes are little islands of cells. These cell clusters are called islet cells. They make substances—hormones—which are released into the bloodstream. The main cells in the islets are beta cells, which make insulin, and alpha cells, which make glucagon (a hormone that increases blood sugar levels, instead of lowering it like insulin). There are also delta cells, which make other hormones, but they are not as important to understanding diabetes.

Our bodies manufacture antibodies, which are special little proteins that attach to and destroy unwanted invaders, such as bacteria. Antibodies protect us from infection and help fight an infection when we do get one. But the body has to be able to distinguish between normal cells and invaders. In type 1 diabetes, the body gets confused and makes a major mistake. For reasons we don't fully understand, the body thinks that its own beta cells are foreign intruders and makes antibodies to attack them. When these antibodies attach to the beta cells they cause the cells to die. Interestingly, these antibodies are so specific that they don't attack the other types of cells in the islets. So the alpha and delta cells are unaffected, at least by this antibody assault.

We can measure the antibodies that are circulating in the blood and destroying beta cells. In children and some adults with type 1 diabetes, at the time of diagnosis and for about six months afterward, tests for islet-cell antibodies can be positive. Antibodies against

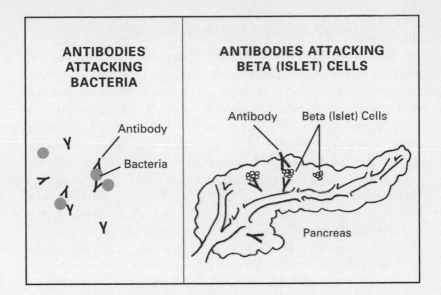

insulin, called anti-insulin antibodies, are also positive, but measuring these is only useful before someone is started on insulin shots.

People don't lose the function of their beta cells all at once, even if it sometimes seems that way. What happens is that the cells are slowly killed off over time. At the point where about half of the beta cells are lost, blood sugar levels start to increase. Sometimes, when someone gets a virus or another illness, they become resistant to the action of insulin. This happens in everyone, but if your beta cells are already partially destroyed your blood sugar levels can climb and you can quickly become quite ill.

Sometimes people must have surgery to remove most or all of the pancreas. This means they lose not only their beta cells, but their alpha cells, too. Such patients wake up from surgery with sudden, very brittle diabetes. These people functionally have a form of type 1 diabetes, although some doctors and reseachers categorize it differently because it isn't due to an autoimmune process.

Latent Autoimmune Diabetes of the Adult (LADA)

We used to think that type 1 diabetes occurred only in children, but now we know that it can happen at any age. When type 1 diabetes starts in adults it begins much more gradually than in children and often can be confused with type 2 diabetes. Adult patients are initially treated with pills, but these tend not to work well and insulin is usually required early on. LADA is sometimes called type 1.5 diabetes, since it can start as a confusing intermediate between type 1 and type 2 diabetes. However, because it involves such a slowly destructive process of the beta cells I prefer to use the term LADA, because I think it best describes what is happening. To test for it we measure the blood for anti-GAD antibodies. Don't worry about the name—GAD stands for glutamic acid decarboxylase and isn't something you need to remember. What you *do* need to remember is that anti-GAD antibodies stay positive for many years, and can be tested at any time to determine if you have LADA. I've had patients who were unsuccessfully treated with pills for a number of years, and then were put on insulin plus pills, with fluctuating and frustrating blood sugar levels. These patients actually were happy to find out that they had positive anti-GAD antibodies and LADA, because it gave them a correct diagnosis, an explanation of why their blood sugar levels had been so difficult to control, and a specific treatment for their diabetes using long-acting insulin (which I'll talk about in chapter 15).

....

"'Don't worry, you can still have cake.'"

This is the story of Zippora Karz, who was a principal ballerina for the New York City Ballet and was diagnosed with type 1 diabetes as a young adult. She was treated incorrectly for a long time because the doctors she saw didn't understand what type of diabetes she had or how to help her balance her needs as a performer with diabetes.

It was 1987, my third year in the New York City Ballet. I was just eighteen years old. The year before, I had been given the role of the Sugar Plum Fairy in The Nutcracker. *Now the director of the com-*

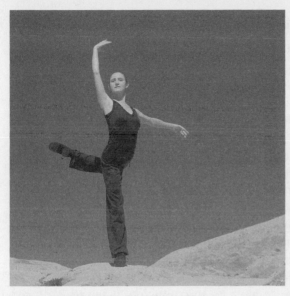

pany was choreographing a new piece and I had one of the leading roles. I was incredibly excited and was working extremely hard every day. But I didn't feel right. I felt more fatigued than I should have and tried to ignore the symptoms that were affecting me daily, from hunger pangs and frequent urination to a spaced-out feeling in my head. But it was the sores under my arms where the costumes rubbed that threatened my ability to perform. They got so infected I could not lift my arms and forced me to go to a doctor.

The doctor checked me out and did some blood tests. Almost right away she told me I had something called diabetes. She said my blood sugar level was 350 and then handed me a number of pamphlets on what could happen to me—heart disease and stroke, blindness, kidney failure, and leg and foot amputations. I was preoccupied with the time. I had to get back to the theater to put on my makeup and get ready for that evening's performance. I asked her what I should do for this diabetes problem. She said I would have to make another appointment so we could discuss how to take insulin. She seemed busy and didn't provide any explanation of what diabetes was or what I was to expect. Before she rushed out of the examination room I asked her what I could do in the meantime and what I should eat. As a dancer I had spent a lot of time working on exercise and diet, and was not a stranger to the world of nutrition. The doctor said, "Don't worry, you can still have cake." Then she left. Since I never ate cake, this comment was not particularly helpful. I sat in the cab back to the theater completely confused and dismayed by what had just happened.

I never went back to that woman. It didn't take me long to realize

I would need more direct answers. I found a doctor that advocated very tight control for maintaining a healthy life with diabetes. Blood sugar checks were frequent, as were tiny amounts of insulin (often in diluted form) to maintain blood sugars as close to normal as possible. Any blood sugar over 120 was to be treated as too high. I didn't know how dangerous this was for me as an athlete performing every night on stage, putting me at high risk for low blood sugar reactions.

I would always check my blood sugar before I went onstage and then adjust my insulin dose. Once, when I had two pieces on the program, I came off after the first piece very frustrated at myself and my body. My head was spacey and I couldn't feel my toes as I tried to dance on the tips of them. I didn't want the company to see me falling apart like this and assume diabetes had altered my promising future. I checked my blood sugar and it was 150. I blamed everything on that and took a shot, which was way too much insulin. By the time the last piece was starting I was on the verge of passing out with a blood sugar of 20. I didn't tell anyone except my sister, who was also in the company. After too many similar events I sought a new doctor.

I next found myself in an office with someone who could not believe what I had been through. This doctor felt my diabetes was not severe enough to require insulin and that I needed to take a break from shots and checking my blood sugars. I started taking pills, put my insulin and my meter away, and went on with my performance schedule.

I thought that this approach was working for me except for the fact that I dropped from 110 to a very gaunt 95 pounds. All of my attempts to appear "unchanged," despite diabetes backfired and the company started to take me out of roles. Pills were obviously not the way to go.

Next I found a doctor who was very balanced in her approach to diabetes. I went back to frequent blood sugar monitoring and taking injections of insulin, but never right before I went onstage. I always kept my meter right offstage in my dance bag and always kept something to reverse a low blood sugar in it. I was finally learning how to adapt to having diabetes.

As I learned the delicate play of dancing with diabetes I also had to look reality in the face. Dancing was my passion, but was this lifestyle realistic for a person with type 1 diabetes? Part of me felt relieved at the idea of quitting. I was tired. But more than that I had lost confidence in my body and in my dancing. Using diabetes as an excuse felt like an easy way out. I thought long and hard about this and eventually decided if I quit then I would never know the truth. So I stayed with the company and hung in there. I eventually found a way to balance my diet, exercise, and performances. Ultimately, I was promoted to the rank of soloist ballerina of the New York City Ballet, where I performed until August 1999.

....

THE CLUES TO TYPE 1 DIABETES

You are more likely to have type 1 diabetes if you are thin, if you've had diabetes since you were a kid, if you are not from a high-risk ethnic group for type 2 diabetes (Latino, African American, Asian American, American Indian, Pacific Islander), and if you don't have a family history of type 2 diabetes. The cases that are more difficult to diagnose are people who develop type 1 diabetes when they are older, in their twenties and upward. Many doctors are used to thinking that all diabetes in adults is type 2 diabetes. But this just isn't true anymore.

By diagnosing people appropriately I know better how to treat them.

I test almost all adult patients who I think might have type 1 diabetes for anti-GAD antibodies and LADA, particularly those who aren't overweight, who have either newly diagnosed diabetes or diabetes that isn't responding easily to pills. One of the reasons I do this is because I tend to get the difficult cases, the ones no one else can figure out. By diagnosing people appropriately I know better how to treat them. When Zippora got diabetes we didn't have this antibody test available. In a way it wasn't needed—Zippora was thin and relatively young and had no risk factors for type 2 diabetes. But the doctor who took her off insulin thought she had type 2 diabetes because she got it as a young adult. He didn't realize that type 1 diabetes can occur at any age.

An even more classic example is my patient Frank. He came to see me after having been diagnosed with type 2 diabetes about six months earlier. He wasn't responding very well to pills (glyburide and metformin). Frank was also the local cop in my neighborhood, so every time he had a question or needed something from me, he would either drive up in front of my house and sound his air horn or he'd pull me over, flashing lights and all, when I was driving home from work (not exactly an office visit—at least not for *me*).

Frank isn't thin; he's a stocky Italian cop, who is in good physical shape. He was in his early fifties when I first met him and had no family history of diabetes. Although looking at him I thought he was a classic patient with type 2 diabetes, I decided to test his antibodies just to be sure. It turned out that he had positive anti-GAD antibodies and was really becoming a person with type 1 diabetes. Over the next year he switched from pills to insulin injections, which he now gives several times per day. Knowing what type of diabetes Frank had allowed me to treat him more quickly and aggressively with insulin, instead of trying different combinations of pills, or pills and insulin.

MAKING THE CASE FOR A SPECIALIST

I think that everyone who has type 1 diabetes should be seen by an endocrinologist who specializes in the care of people with type 1 diabetes. Not everyone will agree with me on this, but type 1 diabetes is fairly uncommon and physicians in general practice may only have one or two patients with type 1 diabetes. Compare that to someone like me, who sees five or six patients with type 1 diabetes every day—that makes for a big difference in experience over the years.

A physician isn't necessarily the best person to be doing a lot of the day-to-day diabetes management—a diabetes educator is often the one who does this best.

Treating someone with type 1 diabetes means interpreting data, reviewing blood sugar levels, adjusting insulin doses, and teaching carbohydrate counting. It means using the newest technology we have available for monitoring and treating the disease. A physician isn't necessarily the best person to be doing a lot of the day-to-day diabetes management—a diabetes educator is often the one who does the best. Normally, someone with a general practice doesn't have an educator in the office, whereas an endocrinologist usually will.

Try to find an endocrinologist you can work with who has a team that includes a diabetes educator and a nutritionist. A good place to find a diabetes team is to go to the American Diabetes Association website (www.diabetes.org) and look for a list of recognized diabetes education programs in your community. They are mostly located in big cities, where there are many people with diabetes, rather than in smaller towns. I have patients who fly in to see me from around the country, because they can't find a good endocrinologist in their community. This can only work if the patient has a good general doctor back home. Everyone needs someone to follow them where they live, someone to go to when they are sick.

Let's say you have new-onset type 1 diabetes and came to see me. Initially I would follow you quite intensively, especially if you were very recently diagnosed. I would see you at least once a week, often with daily e-mails and phone calls in between visits. But after your insulin plan was worked out, and you'd learned and relearned the skills you need to treat your diabetes, your contacts with me and our team would be much less frequent, usually routine follow-up visits every three months to check your A1C level and to keep you updated as to what's happening in the field of diabetes.

Zippora Karz was living and dancing in New York City when she was diagnosed with diabetes. She had access to many endocrinologists and was very persistent in changing doctors until she found one she could work with to help her manage her diabetes and continue dancing. Because of her persistence, Zippora has done amazingly well. She had a successful career in the ballet and is now working as a teacher and performer in Los Angeles. She has no complications from her diabetes and serves as a role model to lots of young people who have diabetes.

....

FIFTEEN

USING INSULIN IN THE TREATMENT OF TYPE 1 DIABETES

To treat type 1 diabetes you need to take insulin shots. I hope that in the future we will have other ways to treat and even cure type 1 diabetes, but for now the only way to get insulin into your body is with injections. If you were to swallow insulin it wouldn't work—the acid in your stomach would destroy it. Other ways of giving insulin, such as inhaled insulin, insulin spray, and special insulin pills, are being researched. But they are not yet available for general use. So for now if you have type 1 diabetes you need to learn about giving yourself insulin shots.

MIMICKING THE BODY'S NORMAL INSULIN ACTIVITY

In someone who doesn't have diabetes, the pancreas is able to make just the right amount of insulin as needed to balance the food that is eaten with the insulin already there. The healthy pancreas makes a little bit of insulin all of the time. We call this the basal insulin. The basal insulin is the amount of insulin you need to make to compensate for the sugar made by your liver. In theory, if you don't eat anything at all the basal insulin level would keep your blood sugar levels constant—neither too high nor too low. Whenever you eat, your blood sugar level goes up. This tells your pancreas to release more insulin. The more carbohydrate (sugar) you eat, the more insulin your body needs to make to compensate. We call this mealtime insulin or bolus insulin. So in someone without diabetes, the body has a low basal level of insulin and releases pre-meal bursts or boluses of insulin. This keeps the blood sugar level normal all day long.

The more carbohydrate (sugar) you eat, the more insulin your body needs to make to compensate.

Someone with type 1 diabetes makes no insulin. So we try to make the insulin shots match what the normal pancreas would do, which means ideally you give yourself a basal insulin and then pre-meal boluses of insulin. The problem is that the closer you try to mimic a normal pancreas, the more often you have to test your blood sugar and give insulin shots. In the old days, we had you give yourself two shots of insulin per day, one before breakfast and one before dinner. These shots were fixed—the doses didn't change. So you had to eat meals with exactly the same composition at exactly the same time each day. Such simple regimens are very limiting because you have to adjust your life around your insulin doses.

My goal is to have you adjust your insulin doses to fit your life. I want you to have the flexibility to eat when and what you want. This is possible with type 1 diabetes, but requires a great deal of diligence on your part, as well as a health care team who can educate you and help you progress. When I first see a patient with type 1 diabetes who hasn't really learned how to master a more flexible regimen, I tell the patient that for the next few weeks it will be a little like diabetes school. Basic concepts and principles of logging, insulin dose adjustments, and carbohydrate counting need to be mastered. I also give patients the choice of insulin delivery—syringes or insulin pens, multiple injections or an insulin pump. I teach the options and let the patient choose what works best for him or her. In my clinic it is the willingness to work at achieving good control that leads to good outcomes; it is not one device or another that is the answer. Whatever the chosen approach, it needs to be followed consistently, ideally in conjunction with our health care team, who can interpret results and help reach goals.

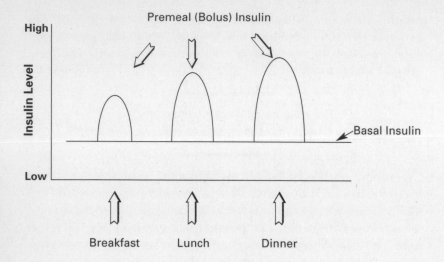

Premeal (Bolus) Insulin

Basal Insulin

Insulin Level — High / Low

Breakfast   Lunch   Dinner

INSULIN TYPES

To understand using insulin you need to know the various types of insulin that are available. In the old days, most insulin came from animal sources, generally pigs or cows. Now, nearly all insulin is laboratory-made to be identical to human insulin. So unless you specifically ask for something different, you get a form of synthetic human insulin.

The most basic form of human insulin is regular insulin. This insulin is clear in color and is just like the insulin that comes from your pancreas. The problem with regular insulin is that it forms clumps under your skin after you inject it, and these clumps slow down how quickly it gets absorbed. To get around this absorption problem, drug companies changed the structure of the insulin a little bit, so it is absorbed more reliably and more quickly (or slowly, as I'll explain). These insulin molecules are called insulin analogues and have really revolutionized my ability to treat people with type 1 diabetes. This is because analogues allow me to more closely approximate normal insulin secretion in my patients.

Humalog (lispro) and Novolog (aspart) are the two rapid-acting insulin analogues. After you inject them, they start to work really quickly, which is the way a normal pancreas would function. Lantus (glargine) is a long-acting insulin analogue, which stay in the body as a steady, basal insulin. Almost all of my patients with type 1 diabetes are on some combination of these fast and slow insulin analogues.

The older preparations of insulin work less well. When regular insulin is mixed with something called protamine it becomes cloudy and is absorbed more slowly. This is called NPH insulin. When regular insulin is mixed with acetate crystals it becomes lente and ultralente insulins, which are more slow-acting than regular insulin. Some people really like these older insulins, and I don't tend to switch people if they are doing well on them. But when patients are having problems I often help them by switching them to insulin analogues.

Mixtures of insulin exist and are useful if you don't vary your insulin doses and lifestyle. But since most of the people I treat have very active lifestyles and want more flexibility than fixed doses can give, I often change them from premixed to self-mixed insulin. However, if you are using a mixture and are happy with it, have an A1C of less than 7 percent, and experience relatively infrequent episodes of hypoglycemia, then you should stick with it.

CREATING YOUR OWN INSULIN REGIMEN

Injecting Insulin and *Pumping Insulin* are two useful books devoted to teaching you about developing an intensive insulin regimen. Both go through the theory and practical use of intensive insulin regimens and one of the things I find most helpful is that they have worksheets where you can practice figuring out your own insulin doses. Although these books can be helpful, I still think everyone needs a team with a diabetes educator, nutritionist, and physician, all of whom are familiar with treating patients with type 1 diabetes. In addition, in larger cities you often can find support groups to join. However, don't go to a general diabetes support group, where most of the patients will have type 2 diabetes and be on pills. Try to find a support group for people on insulin pumps, which is a form of intensive insulin therapy. That way you can meet with others and discuss their personal experiences with using insulin intensively.

Basal Insulin Doses

As I mentioned above, when you do intensive insulin therapy you will need a basal insulin dose. This can either be given through an insulin pump or with an injection of Lantus insulin. The Lantus insulin is usually given once a day, in the morning or the evening. Some people need to take it twice a day, but most of the time it is a once daily insulin. The dose of Lantus will be figured out by your physician, and will be roughly equal to half of your total daily dose of insulin. In my lean patients with type 1 diabetes the dose is usually somewhere between 10 and 20 units, although the dose can vary and needs to be determined individually.

Bolus Insulin Doses

The Carbohydrate Count

Premeal insulin doses are always based on two factors. The first is a calculation based on how much carbohydrate you are going to eat. This entails totaling how many grams of carbohydrate you are going to eat; if you are used to using the exchange system, then 1 exchange equals 15 grams of carbohydrate. The ratio is adjusted for each person, but we often start with 1 unit of rapid-acting insulin (Humalog or Novolog, given through the pump or by injection) for every 15 grams of carbohydrate (or 1 exchange). So if you are eating two pieces of bread that each equal 15 grams of carbohydrate, you would take 2 units of insulin before the meal.

The Correction Factor

The second part of the bolus insulin equation is a correction factor for what your blood sugar level is before you eat. If your blood sugar level is too low, you give less insulin. If it is too high, you give more insulin. We have you pick a target level, for the moment we'll say 150 mg/dl, and then give extra insulin to get down to that target. We analyze your blood sugar levels and insulin doses to determine what your correction factor is. Let's say that 1 unit of insulin is needed to drop your blood sugar 50 points. That is a correction factor of 50. Therefore, if your blood sugar level is 250 and you want to bring it down to 150, you would give 2 units of insulin (2 units × 50 = a fall of 100 points). This doesn't always work perfectly, but adjusting your insulin using this system allows you to better account for changes in your diet and blood sugar levels.

Adjusting for Exercise

The other adjustment that needs to be made is for exercise or an increase of physical activity. When people exercise, insulin is used more efficiently in their bodies so less is needed. We often have you give less insulin for a meal if you are going to exercise soon after eating. That way, you have less risk of a low blood sugar problem developing later on. Sometimes you may need to give less insulin after you exercise, as well. The best way to determine your insulin needs for exercise is to carefully track your blood sugar levels before and after you exercise for a few days, and then work with your diabetes health care team to figure out what your insulin doses should be.

DEALING WITH HYPOGLYCEMIA

Although I have discussed hypoglycemia in other sections of this book, I want to discuss it more formally here. It is the constant concern of a person with diabetes and a factor that limits our use of insulin in attempting to make blood sugar levels normal. Although we try hard to help patients find the right insulin doses, it is impossible to get it completely right all the time.

Hypoglycemia is defined as a blood sugar level that is below 70 mg/dl. Symptoms associated with hypoglycemia include weakness, shakiness, hunger, rapid heartbeat, all of which go away when some form of rapid-acting carbohydrate is eaten. This sounds simple enough, but sometimes you either don't feel or can't feel the warning signs of hypoglycemia. You can start to lose consciousness and go into a coma if hypoglycemia is not reversed. We call the common warning signs of hypoglycemia the adrenergic symptoms. They are signs that your body has released catecholamines (norepinephrine and epinephrine) into your bloodstream to help raise your blood sugar level.

If you lose your adrenergic symptoms, either because you've had diabetes for a long time or because you often have low blood sugar levels, you only have the neuroglycopenic symptoms. This means that instead of having a warning sign you start to lose consciousness or slur your words or start losing your vision, all because your brain is not getting enough sugar. Since your brain can only use sugar to function, if you fall below a certain level your brain stops working correctly. These serious low blood sugar episodes (called severe hypoglycemic reactions) usually require someone else to help you recover from them, either by injecting you with glucagon or getting you to drink some juice or calling 911. It's important to avoid these severe reactions, because if they happen, for example, when you are driving you could crash, or they could cause you to fall over or to have seizures, among other serious problems.

Hypoglycemic reactions happen for a variety of reasons. A common cause is missing a meal or snack, or eating less carbohydrate than you think you will. Alcohol can cause hypoglycemia. Exercise can increase the risk for hypoglycemia for twelve hours or more after activity because your body becomes more sensitive to the effects of insulin. But we don't always know why hypoglycemia episodes occur, especially those that come on in the middle of the night.

**Exercise can cause hypoglycemia that can occur
for twelve hours or more after activity.**

Treating diabetes is a real balancing act. When you are on an intensive insulin regimen, expect that you will have two or three mild low blood sugar reactions per week. If you can't sense low blood sugar reactions, however, and have frequent severe low reactions, your doctor might raise your target blood sugar levels and try to prevent you from having any low reactions at all. I can often help a person regain their sense of low blood sugar levels by rais-

ing their overall blood sugar levels for a while. It se
sugar levels are too low too often your body acc
and stops sensing your falling blood sugar levels.
term for this—hypoglycemia-induced autonomic fa
enough to know that too many lows cause you to lc
to sense lows, and that raising your blood sugar levels for a while
can remedy the situation.

Treating Mild Low Blood Sugar Reactions

Treating mild low blood sugar levels is something of an art. Most
people hate the feeling of having a low blood sugar reaction and
want to use it as an excuse to eat everything they usually don't,
such as candy, soda, and cake. But if you eat too much sugar, your
blood sugar levels will skyrocket up again and then you will be in
the situation of swinging low and high and low again. We teach
people the *Rule of 15:* If your blood sugar is 50 to 70 mg/dl eat 15
grams of fast-acting carbohydrate, wait 15 minutes, and recheck your
blood sugar. If it is above 70 and you're feeling better, that's fine.
If it hasn't come up, eat 15 grams more of carbohydrate. If your
blood sugar is below 50, eat 30 grams of carb at first and follow the
steps above.

Examples of 15 grams of simple carbohydrate include 3 glucose
tablets, ½ cup (4 ounces) juice, ½ can sugary soda, 6 LifeSavers,
1 cup (8 ounces) milk, 2 tablespoons of table sugar, 1 tablespoon
of honey, or 1 tube of glucose gel.

This may seem easy enough, but problems happen if you don't
have any fast-acting carbohydrate with you and have to lose time
trying to find some. Part of living well with diabetes is being prepared. When you have type 1 diabetes, always having some form of
simple, fast-acting carbohydrate with you is a necessity.

Usually after you treat a low blood sugar reaction we suggest that
you eat a snack containing fat, protein, and carbohydrate within
half an hour or so, or eat the meal that comes next. That way
you'll have enough longer-acting carbohydrate in you to prevent
your blood sugar levels from falling again.

Treating Severe Low Blood Sugar Reactions

If you have a severe reaction and can't treat your low blood sugar reaction yourself, it is best to have someone give you an injection of glucagon. Glucagon is never something you give yourself—it is for when you are not able to treat yourself. Glucagon is sort of an anti-insulin and raises your blood sugar level fairly rapidly. Many people forget to keep glucagon in their refrigerator and since it expires every six months or so, you have to keep getting more even if you don't use it. It's completely understandable to forget about glucagon, especially if you never use it. But it is still something you should try to keep around if you live with someone who could give it to you if you needed it.

Glucagon is never something you give yourself—it is for when you are not able to treat yourself.

If glucagon isn't available, 911 should be called so that you can receive immediate help. The paramedics have glucagon, as well as intravenous sugar that they can give you. The worst thing someone can do, on the other hand, is to try to force you to drink juice when you are not conscious. You could inhale the juice into your lungs and that could cause serious problems. On the other hand, gently rubbing cake icing gel or pure maple syrup onto your gums might help bring your blood sugar level up a bit. The person doing this just needs to be sure that they aren't at risk for being bitten.

In case you have a severe low blood sugar reaction when you are alone, it is very important that you wear a medical alert bracelet. There are many companies that make medical alert products; here are some websites to check out: www.medicalert.org, www.americanmedical-id.com, www.medic-id.com, and www.911med411.com. Some companies also make nontraditional-looking medical alerts that are particularly good for children. (I like them, too.) Some examples are at these websites: www.missbrooke.com and www.laurenshope.com. At the website www.childrenwithdiabetes.com a fairly complete listing of all of the medical alert providers is available.

TOOLS FOR INJECTING INSULIN

Although we can't cure diabetes yet, the tools for managing diabetes are becoming more and more refined. You'll want to keep up on what is available because many of these devices can help you manage your diabetes more easily and may hurt less to use. A good place to look is in the patient-focused publication of the ADA called *Diabetes Forecast*. Each year they publish a new "Diabetes Product Guide" that runs through all of the tools available for treating diabetes and where to buy them.

Syringes

Simple things may make a big difference. For instance, insulin syringes come in a variety of sizes—some hold only 30 units and offer half-unit increments to make measuring small doses easier. Needle size can vary. The smaller syringes often have the thinnest needles; most people prefer insulin syringes that have short needles. Needle size is listed as a number, a gauge, and the larger the gauge, the smaller the needle. Currently the smallest needle is a 30-gauge needle. In order to get these syringes your doctor needs to write the prescription very carefully. I state the brand of insulin syringe I want (often BD), the capacity of the syringe (30 units, 50 units, 100 units), if I want ½-unit increments (only available on the 30-unit size), the length of the needle (often short), and sometimes I even put the gauge, all this to be sure the pharmacist knows exactly what syringe you should be given.

Insulin Pens

Insulin pens are wonderful devices that literally look like thick pens. They contain insulin and you select your dose by turning a dial. The benefit of pens is that you don't have to worry about the fuss and bother of drawing up insulin from a vial with a syringe—you have a prefilled pen all ready to go. Some pens are completely disposable and some pens have replaceable cartridges. Either way, once you put a pen needle on the top of the pen you are ready to use it.

With all pens you need to flush a new needle with insulin the first time you attach it. Otherwise, you will be giving less insulin than you thought with the first injection. Usually 4 to 5 units is enough to flush the needle—just watch for insulin squirting out of the end of the needle so you know that you've flushed it adequately. Then dial the dose you want to give, insert the needle into your skin, and push the plunger down. Wait for five seconds after the insulin is injected before you remove it from your skin.

These pens are easy to carry in your purse or backpack and are helpful when you are giving insulin injections before each meal. The downside to pens is that you can't mix insulins. They also have a limit of how much insulin they can give in one dose—this is generally around 60 units. If you require more insulin you will have to give several shots. Finally, pens are often not paid for by insurance companies. Even though every insurance company executive I know finds it easier to give insulin with a pen than with a needle and syringe, items that are primarily for convenience (such as pens) are rarely covered. In some cases, for example if you have decreased vision or an impairment of your nerves or muscles that makes drawing up insulin particularly difficult or if your employer or school doesn't let you bring in syringes, pens can be covered.

Insulin Pumps

I have lots of patients who use insulin pumps. I think that insulin pump therapy is harder to use than multiple injections because the pumps have to be babied a bit. But I have patients who absolutely love their insulin pumps and would never part with them. I have other patients who tried an insulin pump and quickly went back to shots. This is fine—no one therapy is right for everyone.

If you decide to try a pump it is not the same as permanently altering some part of your body. A pump is a mechanical device, about the size of a pager, which releases a constant flow of rapid-acting insulin through a catheter that is inserted under your skin. A pump does *not* measure your blood sugar levels—you still have to prick your finger for that. But it does deliver a slow little trickle of insulin based on a basal rate that you figure out with your health care team. It also can deliver insulin in larger single doses. Before you eat you push a button and get a dose (the bolus we discussed earlier) of insulin. You don't have to give an injection before each meal—you simply give it through your pump. In some ways this is much more convenient than shots—the insulin is ready to give, right in the pump. But there are several things that make this system difficult. For one thing you have to wear the pump somewhere on your body. Men tend to wear it on their belts; women will often hide it in their bra. At night you have to find some way to deal with the pump—boxer shorts or a pajama top with a pocket tend to work well. Tubing is also a part of the device as is a catheter needle. The tubing connects the pump to the catheter, which, of course, you constantly have to keep inserted under your skin for the pump to function.

A pump is a mechanical device, about the size of a pager, which releases a constant flow of rapid-acting insulin through a catheter that is inserted under your skin.

The pump catheter needs to be reinserted every two to three days. Many of the catheters have devices that are designed to help with insertion. Without them, you just sort of jam it under your skin. You have to be taught how to use the pump; you have to deal with it quite carefully because you don't want to increase your risk for getting an infection.

The other thing you *must* do while on the pump is to test your blood sugar levels at least four times a day. This is because the tubing that carries the insulin is very thin and sometimes a clog or a kink can disrupt insulin flow from the pump. Often the way you know this is happening is because your blood sugar level is going up too high. If you don't catch the problem early it can become serious and you can go into ketoacidosis (a serious metabolic crisis that can happen to people with type 1 diabetes if they don't get enough insulin). What I suggest is that if the blood sugar level is above 350 mg/dl, you give insulin with the pump and wait for an hour. Then you retest. If your blood sugar level is not falling in response to the insulin, then you have to assume that the pump is not working correctly, and you should be ready to give insulin by injection to keep yourself out of trouble.

The newer pumps have all sorts of great features. Blood sugar levels can be sent from your blood sugar meter into the pump through an infrared signal. Newer pumps also have dose calculators so that if you input your blood sugar reading and your carbohydrate intake, the pump will figure out how much insulin you need to take. These pumps are very good at determining doses, but they are only as accurate as you are at carbohydrate counting. Data from such pumps can be downloaded into a computer for complete analysis of blood sugar levels and insulin dosing.

You shouldn't even try the pump unless you are willing and able to test your blood sugars at least four times a day without fail.

Unlike long-acting insulin shots, which give you a fairly constant amount of insulin, the pump allows you to make very small changes in the basal rate in order to cover changing insulin needs during the day and particularly overnight. Pumps also are easily turned off—operation can be suspended or the basal rate reduced if you are exercising or your blood sugar levels drop too low. This capability for easy on and off—the best part of the insulin pump—is also what makes using it more risky than shots. When it's off you don't have a steady basal flow or any long-acting insulin in your system to smooth things out or keep you safe.

People often ask me if they have to be attached to the pump all of the time. The answer is that you can take it off for brief periods, but it really needs to stay on your body most of the time. Some people hate the idea of being attached to something all the time; others don't mind at all. The best person to talk to about pumps may be someone who has been on a pump and has practical experience with it. If you choose to start on a pump, make sure you have a good teacher to answer all of your questions.

We used to put people in the hospital to start them on insulin pumps, but not anymore. Everything is done in an outpatient setting. But in the first days after you start on the pump you need to talk to your diabetes educator daily, so the doses can be adjusted and you can be safely taught how to troubleshoot the pump. Again, I need to stress that you shouldn't even try the pump unless you are willing and able to test your blood sugars at least four times a day without fail. Anything less could prove disastrous.

DEVICES FOR MEASURING BLOOD SUGAR LEVELS

Meters

Meters are battery-powered devices used to test blood sugar level. New models of meters are coming out all the time—meters that are smaller, faster, and require smaller drops of blood. Some of them have self-contained blood test strips, some have memories where you can input information about your insulin doses and lifestyle, and some even have alarms to remind you to test your blood sugar levels.

Since the new meters are often better than old meters, at least once a year you should show your diabetes health care provider your meter and ask if it is up-to-date or if you should get a newer model. Often you will be given a meter—I have lots of free meters to give away in my office. The meter companies make most of their money on the disposable blood test strips, not the meters, so you can easily get a new meter free or inexpensively. But before you change meters, be sure to check that your insurance company will pay for the strips of the meter you choose. Some insurance plans limit you to certain meter brands.

Be sure to check that your insurance company will pay for the strips of the meter you choose.

If possible, you should bring your meter to your doctor visit and compare its results to a blood sample measured in the office. Most meters come with calibration solutions that can help you make sure your meter is functioning properly. The most important things you can do to make sure your meter will give you accurate information is to keep it clean and to make sure your strips are not expired and are kept in a closed container. The strips are the most fragile part of the system, and exposure to air or heat can change how they work. You also need to make sure the code shown on your meter matches the code on your strips. Each time you open a new vial of strips you will need to change the code on your meter. (Some meters do this automatically and others require that you enter the code yourself.)

Most people prick a fingertip to get a drop of blood for testing. I have had some trouble with people using forearm (instead of fingertip) testing. Forearm testing is only accurate if your blood sugar level is stable, that is, not rising or falling. Unfortunately, if you have lost your ability to sense low blood sugar reactions, you may not be able to tell if your blood sugar levels are rising or falling before you choose to poke your forearm or your fingertips. This can lead to falsely high blood sugar readings and some of my more brittle patients with type 1 diabetes have gone way too low relying on this type of testing. So if in doubt, use your fingertips.

Monitoring Devices

Monitoring your blood sugar levels by pricking your finger before meals gives you only a tiny fraction of the information you need to understand how your blood sugar levels are fluctuating throughout the day. Since I became a diabetes specialist I have been eagerly awaiting the development of monitors that can continuously test your blood sugar levels. These monitors would let you know, just by looking at a pagerlike device, what your blood sugar level is at any time of the day or night. But even more important, a continuous monitor could alert you if your blood sugar level were falling too low or rising too high. It could also show patterns. For instance, if your blood sugar level before a meal is 100 mg/dl and falling quickly you may need to give a much smaller dose of insulin than if your blood sugar is 100 and rising rapidly.

Being able to adjust to all of this information is one concern about using continuous monitors. It could be dangerous to give yourself insulin every few minutes because your blood sugar level is high, instead of giving insulin once and then waiting an hour or two to see how your body responds. Giving too much insulin too often can also be quite dangerous. On the other hand, the added benefit of being alerted to rising and falling blood sugar levels seems worth the risk and the training needed to use continuous monitors safely.

In order to get around the problem of overreacting to blood sugar levels (and the problems we have had with accuracy) the first sensor, the Medtronic MiniMed CGMS (Continuous Glucose Monitoring System), does not allow you to see the blood sugar levels it is measuring. Instead, it records the blood sugar levels into a small black box that is attached to you, which is downloaded after three days of use so your health care team can look at your blood sugar levels. This form of historical analysis can be helpful at identifying patterns, but it is not as useful as knowing blood sugar levels in real time. The next version of the CGMS should include high and low alerts, but the problem in development has been making sure these devices read blood sugar levels accurately. They don't measure your blood the same way you do when you stick your finger. They are inserted under your skin into the fat tissue there. What they are reading is called the interstitial fluid, a clear fluid that bathes the cells in your body. Sugar goes in and out of your interstitial fluid just as it goes in and out of the blood, but the results from testing it have to be interpreted differently to make them correspond to blood sugar levels we are used to seeing.

The Glucowatch Biographer is the first real-time continuous monitor. It looks like an oversized watch and you generally wear it on your wrist, although you can attach it to other parts of your body as well. It sends a little electric current into your skin, which lets it draw up fluid into the monitor. It reads your blood sugar level every ten minutes. The problems with the Glucowatch right now are many: it is hard to wear and use, the results often aren't accurate, it only works for about twelve hours at a time, and it has to be warmed up for an hour or two before using. Many people find that it irritates their skin. For these reasons, and because it isn't a replacement for fingertip blood sugar level monitoring, it isn't used widely. On the other hand, for some patients who are worried about having low blood sugar reactions overnight, it can be very comforting to have an alarm to warn them.

Other, more effective, continuous sensors are also being developed. One sensor uses a patch on your arm that sends sugar readings to a pagerlike device. This system will be able to tell you your blood sugar levels every few minutes. The patch lasts for three days and then needs to be changed. Another type of sensor is a little pellet that is surgically inserted under your skin. This pellet will last from six months to a year or two and also sends frequent blood sugar readings to a pagerlike device.

The most ambitious and perhaps most accurate device is one made by Medtronic MiniMed; it is a sensor, like a pacemaker sensor, that is surgically placed into the big blood vessel going to your heart (the superior vena cava). This little sensor reads sugar levels in your blood, not in your interstitial fluid, and because it is continuously being washed over by blood as it empties into your heart, it is very accurate. This type of sensor is being used to measure blood sugar levels in Medtronic MiniMed's complete closed loop system, where patients have a pump implanted into their abdomen. The implanted sensor talks to the pump and insulin doses are given accordingly, similar to the functioning of a normal pancreas. This system is still experimental, but it does work. Hopefully someday we'll have these highly accurate sensors available for more general use.

....

"I don't have to live life thinking that no one cares about me."

Hannah is a sweet waif of a girl who showed up in my office one Monday afternoon with her young mother, Kathleen. Hannah is twelve years old, the age of my son, and had moved to Los Angeles from Ohio. Moving to Los Angeles had been rough on Hannah. She had to leave her circle of friends behind, but perhaps even more than that, she had to leave her beloved horse. She now lives in the middle of Los Angeles, surrounded not by the rolling hills of the Midwest, but by concrete. She feels lonely and angry, and a little bit sad. She currently manages her diabetes with a combination of an insulin pump plus an injection of Lantus, a long-acting insulin.

I was diagnosed with diabetes when I was only six years old. Ever since then my life has been completely different. It has forced me to be

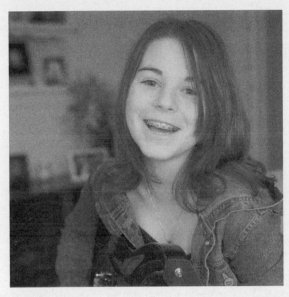

more mature than my friends, and to be aware of the foods that I'm putting into my body. People always say how they feel sorry for me and how it must suck to have to take shots. Of course it does. No one wants to have to take shots and poke their fingers, but it's really not all bad. In a way, it has helped my life. I know more about the human body than most people I know. Growing up with diabetes is very difficult, but it has some benefits.

"Did you check your sugar? Did you take your insulin? Did you take your Lantus?" These are just a few things I hear from people all the time, especially my mom. As much as I hate that people are always bothering me about it, I've come to realize that I need them. Before I moved to California I had a ton of freedom with what I ate and how I took care of myself. My mom hardly ever asked if I did everything I was supposed to do because she trusted me. But lately I've been kind of slacking off, and my mom has gotten down on me for it. It's bothering me because I'm not used to it. And since I'm not used to it, I'm having a hard time letting her help me. Seven years of diabetes has already gotten to me. I sometimes wonder how I'm going to get through the rest of my life.

But my family and friends are amazing. My A1C has been really high for about a year now, but with the help of my family and friends, it has come down to about 9 percent already. That's the great thing about growing up with diabetes; I don't have to live life thinking that no one cares about me. I know that people care because every time my sugar goes too high or too low my friends know what to do, and they don't mind helping. They would gladly give me a sip of their juice, or *their last piece of candy. Some of my friends have even offered to put the insulin into the pump for me when my blood glucose is extremely high. Before moving to California I didn't know what to do with myself. I thought, "Why live? What's the point if I can't even enjoy myself?" Well, guess what? I'm now enjoying myself and having the time of my life. It's people like Dr. Peters, my mom, and of course my friends who make living with diabetes worth all the trouble.*

....

TREATING LATENT AUTOIMMUNE DIABETES OF THE ADULT (LADA)

Everything I've discussed above holds true for treating most people with type 1 diabetes, but treating people with LADA is slightly different. When you have LADA you are slowly losing your beta cells. Because this process is so slow, for a long time it may look as though you have type 2 diabetes—in other words, a combination of insulin resistance plus insulin deficiency instead of insulin deficiency alone. Therefore, for a while you may respond to the oral medications for treating type 2 diabetes. The problem with this is that it may make you worse more quickly. When you have LADA, or any type of newly diagnosed type 1 diabetes, what you want is to keep as many of your beta cells around as possible. The more beta cells you have, the easier your diabetes is to treat, because you aren't completely dependent on getting insulin from shots.

When you have LADA, or any type of newly diagnosed type 1 diabetes, what you want is to keep as many of your beta cells around as possible.

Giving insulin shots helps rest your beta cells and keeps them functioning longer, particularly when compared to drugs that push on your beta cells to make more insulin, like the sulfonylurea agents. So if you have LADA what I recommend is that you start giving yourself a basal insulin as soon as possible—usually a once-a-day injection of Lantus. This dose is often extremely small, around 4 to 10 units (as opposed to the 45 units or more needed in type 2 diabetes). You should adjust the dose of the basal insulin to keep your fasting blood sugar at 100 mg/dl. Then you should test your blood sugar levels before meals and give small doses, often 2 to 4 units of a rapid-acting insulin (Humalog or Novolog) if your premeal blood sugar level is high or you're going to eat extra carbohydrate.

I've had patients who had LADA but didn't know it who were really struggling to treat their diabetes with pills. They found that their blood sugar levels became really well controlled with just a little bit of insulin every day. And although the beta cells eventually will stop working completely, I've had patients go for five years or more with this simpler, effective approach to treating their diabetes.

LOOKING AHEAD

Type 1 diabetes is a simple disease in theory, but a difficult disease to actually treat. It is hard to replace insulin from outside the body, to make up for what your pancreas should be producing. But I have found that my patients can do an amazingly good job living with type 1 diabetes.

There are always going to be things that will be more of a hassle for people with diabetes than for people without diabetes. We've already discussed strategies for ordering meals in unfamiliar restaurants. Travel, especially business travel, can be problematic because your time is not necessarily your own. You have to plan ahead to deal with how injection and meal schedules will be affected by time zone changes, airline meal service (or lack thereof), or overlong meetings and appointments. (Tip: Always carry at least of couple of protein bars or packaged snacks just in case meals are inordinately delayed.) Foreign and adventure travel are even more challenging; be sure to pack copies of prescriptions and to have backup supplies (additional insulin, syringes, blood test strips, and an extra battery for your meter). Even buying over-the-counter cold and cough remedies at your neighborhood pharmacy can be daunting, with their package warnings for people with diabetes. (By the way, most of these warnings have to do with the sugar content of the medications, but it's still a good idea to consult your doctor about them.)

But with all these challenges life with diabetes can be full and satisfying and exciting—even if maybe a bit less spontaneous. A key element to success is to have a supportive diabetes team to help you manage your diabetes as your life changes, from school to work to getting married and having babies and eventually growing old. Your team (and you, yourself, if you don't have such a team) can help you plan for trips as well as keep you updated on the latest developments in the treatment of type 1 diabetes, from newer types of insulin to the latest technologies for monitoring and insulin delivery.

A key element to success is to have a supportive diabetes team to help you manage your diabetes as your life changes, from school to work to getting married and having babies and eventually growing old.

The more you are willing to test your blood sugar and adjust your insulin doses, the more freedom you will have and the better your control will be. All of the testing and adjusting is obviously something of a burden, but it is far better to do it than to suffer the consequences, both immediate and delayed, of poorly controlled diabetes. I am hopeful that within the next ten years our increasing ability to monitor type 1 diabetes and give insulin will make type 1 diabetes a much easier disease to live with. I still hold hope that I will see a cure in my lifetime, as well. But there are no guarantees of a cure. So, for now at least, I have to keep working hard to help you use the existing tools to effectively control your diabetes.

It is my passion, and my mission.

SIXTEEN

PREGNANCY AND THE TREATMENT OF TYPE 1 DIABETES

One of the happiest things I do is to help women with diabetes through their pregnancies. Whenever I meet a new young female patient with diabetes I discuss pregnancy. Often women with diabetes feel that they can't go through a pregnancy and for many that is simply wrong. It definitely takes more work to go through pregnancy when you have diabetes, but of the many mothers I've helped I don't think there is one who would say it wasn't worth it. Yana's story shows the struggle and joy of being pregnant with type 1 diabetes.

"I am the luckiest mom and luckiest woman with diabetes in the world."

Pregnancy was the best thing that ever happened to me. I guess I always knew I wanted to have children, but there are many fears that come to mind when you are a woman who has had type 1 diabetes for twenty-five years and has a lot of diabetic baggage. I wondered: Will I be able to control my sugars? Will my baby suffer the consequences of my diabetes? Will I wind up with a C-section? All are valid fears. But I was saved by planning.

After marrying Robert in 1999 we began to think about becoming parents. The first step was getting my diabetes under control. I chose an insulin pump, but I had a hard time learning how to live with it. It felt like a constant reminder that I was a woman with diabetes; something I didn't often want to remember. Then there's the carb counting. I thought, "Forget it. Who the hell wants to keep records? Can't I just live in denial?" Then I had to refocus my energy on my

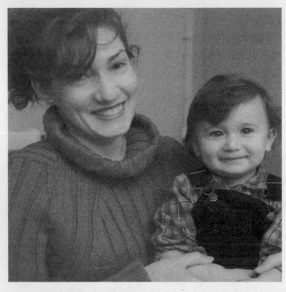

goal—a healthy baby.

First I got used to the pump. Then I got my A1C down to an all-time low of 7 percent! But at my pre-pregnancy eye exam I was shocked to find out that I had diabetic damage in both eyes. I couldn't believe I had retinopathy at age thirty. Dr. Schwartz, my eye doctor, told me that if I didn't take care of my eyes before pregnancy I could lose my eyesight. I couldn't even begin to imagine what that would be like. After many laser surgeries and amazing care I was in the clear.

During that time I switched my diabetes care to Dr. Peters and her team. Working with them I got my A1C to 5.5 percent—in the normal range. So with my sugars under control and my eye problems resolved I was given the green light to start trying to get pregnant. After several nerve-wracking months during which I thought I might be infertile, I discovered I was pregnant. Robert's and my dream of creating a family together was coming true. But now I had to be even more careful. I increased my testing frequency, thought twice about whatever I put into my mouth, and was always worried about pump failure.

When I was three months pregnant my fears were actualized and I had a pump set failure. I was at work and did not have my extra pump changing kit with me. I was so upset at myself. I was worried that my actions and this failure would hurt my baby. My husband came over with a kit and helped me change the pump infusion set. I was so upset that I could not see anything through my tears. To think that my diabetes was hurting this little being that had not yet seen the light of day was overwhelming. The hard part is that you don't know anything for sure until you give birth and that was a long way away.

But on the whole, my pregnancy was amazing. I was going to the doctor's office every week and working with my diabetes team, who treated me with warmth, respect, and great care. My insulin require-ments were steadily increasing throughout the pregnancy and I had to rely more on my husband Robert to help me deal with my insulin pump. Time flew by and before I knew it I was a month away from delivery. I now had to go in weekly to my OB for fetal monitoring tests. After two weeks I was told my baby seemed a little bigger than normal and that if I wanted to have a vaginal delivery I would have to be in-duced. I didn't want to be induced. I was very upset. I felt like the whole experience of feeling the first contractions, packing the bags, and heading to the hospital in the middle of the night was being taken away from me. But I had to get over myself and think of the baby. So I had the amnio, waited for my parents to fly in from New York, and went to the hospital at 4:30 AM to have a baby!

My diabetes team had prepared me for what to do during and after delivery, and what to expect about insulin requirements while breast-feeding. During labor they called the hospital frequently. My mother and husband were at my side during the whole process. I was started on a pitocin drip at 6 AM, got an epidural at 12:30 PM, and by 4:30 PM I was ready to push. I worked very hard for two hours. At one point I saw the doctor looking at the nurse, saying, "I don't know how long we can do this." Suddenly, something bigger than me took over and within ten minutes I pushed my baby out.

Benjamin Adam Nackman was born on Thursday, November 7, 2002, at 8 pounds, 3 ounces, and 20 inches long. They put him on my chest and I held him in my arms. I was in shock. Here was my baby, healthy and normal. He had all ten fingers and all ten toes and he made the most beautiful crying sounds I've heard.

He was checked by the nurses and pediatricians to make sure that his sugars were in the normal range. He had to spend an extra day in the hospital, but Benjamin was a trooper and two days later we were sent home. He is such a gift and a blessing for Robert and me, and our families. I am the luckiest mom and the luckiest woman with dia-betes in the world. I am now planning for round two.

....

PREPARING FOR PREGNANCY

The first rule, as Yana's story attests, is to plan your pregnancy. Your blood sugar level at the time you conceive is important to the healthy development of the baby, so you'll want at least three months if not more to get ready. Here's a basic checklist I go through with my patients before they try to get pregnant:

1. Have your eyes examined by your ophthalmologist. Unfortunately, pregnancy can make diabetic eye disease worse. In a very few of my patients their eye disease was so bad that they were advised not to become pregnant (or risk going blind). Most women do fine, but need to be checked every three months during their pregnancy to be sure no problems develop.

2. Have blood and urine tests to check your kidney function. Even patients with mild kidney damage can have healthy pregnancies. Kidney function may get slightly worse during pregnancy, but returns to the level it was before pregnancy once the baby is born. However, if you have more severe kidney damage, your kidney function could become permanently worse during pregnancy. This is something you should talk over with your kidney specialist. I have never had a patient experience new problems with kidney function during or after pregnancy, but you need to check.

3. Stop or change all drugs that shouldn't be used in pregnancy. This list is long, but does include Lantus insulin, which should not be used during pregnancy. If you are taking Lantus you will need to switch to NPH or an insulin pump and stabilize your blood sugar levels prior to pregnancy. If you are taking oral medications for diabetes you will need to switch to insulin. Other drugs people with diabetes often take are statins (for cholesterol) and ACE inhibitors or ARBs, for high blood pressure—these drugs must be stopped and switched to something safe for pregnancy *before* you get pregnant. Thyroid hormone is safe and required during pregnancy if you are taking it, but you

should have your levels tested before and during pregnancy to be sure they stay normal.

4. Make sure your heart is functioning normally. Not to alarm you, but heart disease is the one thing that can cause a mother to die during pregnancy. Most women of childbearing age don't have any problems with their hearts, but be sure you ask.

5. Treat your blood pressure aggressively. High blood pressure during pregnancy can cause serious problems and requires different medications than it does when you are not pregnant.

6. Be *sure* that your A1C level is less than 7 percent before you become pregnant. The risk of deformities in your baby goes way up if your blood sugar levels are too high. This is not to say that 100 percent of babies will have problems if your sugar levels are elevated, but who wants to risk it? During pregnancy is the one time when your body is responsible for the health of two people. Keep both of you well.

7. Take folic acid supplements (1 mg or more) for several months before you try to get pregnant, to help prevent spinal defects in your baby (this applies whether or not you have diabetes).

THE PREGNANCY TIMELINE

Once you are pregnant you need to be followed by a health care team familiar with treating diabetes in pregnancy. Sometimes this will be your obstetrician, but I prefer to treat my patients myself. Early in pregnancy your insulin requirements will fall; later in pregnancy they will go up and up because insulin resistance increases. Immediately after you deliver, your insulin requirements plummet and then gradually go back up again to your pre-pregnancy needs. Finally, breast-feeding will change your insulin and calorie requirements, as will the lack of sleep.

You will need to be seen by your health care team weekly during your pregnancy. I often substitute faxed blood sugar records alternating with weekly visits, but it really depends on the patient.

Remember, you may be familiar with your body and your diabetes, but you've never experienced the changes brought on by pregnancy before. Those of us who have treated patients with diabetes who are pregnant can provide you with the benefit of our experience. A healthy baby—and mother—is everyone's goal.

....

SEVENTEEN

THE BENEFITS OF CARBOHYDRATE COUNTING

If you learn how to count carbohydrates you will live with type 1 diabetes as successfully as possible. You need to train yourself to do what the beta cells in your pancreas do naturally—guess the amount your blood sugar will rise with a meal then inject just the right amount of insulin to bring your blood sugar back down to normal after you've finished eating. The normal pancreas is so amazing that blood sugar levels never rise above 140 mg/dl, even after eating lots of carbohydrate, such as pancakes with syrup and orange juice.

To learn how to count carbohydrates accurately, you need to study as if you were taking a class in healthy eating. It may take several months to get good at carb counting, but many of my patients have become experts at it.

Carbohydrates are the parts of our food that break down most readily to sugar in our bloodstream; we also use the word to refer to specific foods that have a high proportion of carbohydrates in them. Simple, refined sugars like table sugar are absorbed quickly into the bloodstream and raise glucose levels. More complex sugars, often called starches, have to be broken down before they are absorbed; pasta, rice, bread, and potatoes are rich in these. A patient came to me a few years ago and said he'd read that he should just avoid eating anything white. White foods, with the exception of egg whites and some types of fat, are sugars and starches, and will raise your blood sugar levels if you eat them. Fruits, vegetables, and milk also are sources of carbohydrate.

*Although a high-protein diet is often a good way
to lose weight, in the long term it is important
to have a healthy balance.*

Of course, eating isn't just about carbohydrates, although carbs have the most immediate effect on your blood sugar levels. You want to eat a variety of healthy foods that are high in fiber, vitamins, and high-quality nutrients. You also should try to limit the amount of saturated fat, trans fat, and cholesterol in your diet as much as possible. Although a high-protein diet is often a good way to lose weight, in the long term it is important to have a healthy balance.

The best person to help you with your meal plan is a nutritionist (dietitian) who specializes in helping people with diabetes. He or she can help you find the right foods for your tastes and then learn to count carbohydrates so you can match your insulin dose to the food you eat. The goal is to create a diet that allows you to feel free to have the foods you like, in appropriate quantities, and to give the necessary amount of insulin to cover the blood sugar rise following any meal.

LEARNING CARBOHYDRATE COUNTING

For nearly everyone it takes a lot of practice to learn to be good at carbohydrate counting. You will need at least three tools. The first is a good guide to carbohydrates, such as *Barbara Kraus' Calories and Carbohydrates* or a series of books on carbohydrate counting available from the American Diabetes Association—*Complete Guide to Carb Counting; Diabetes Carbohydrate and Fat Gram Guide;* and *Fast Facts Series: Carb Counting Made Easy* (www.diabetes.org). The second is a food measuring scale, so you can measure your food at home often enough to get a visual image of what 15 grams of rice or pasta looks like. The third is a set of measuring cups. Weight Watchers has a great set of measuring cups that are like scoops; they, too, can really help you learn how to visualize portion size accurately. Once you have your tools, you need to start making simple meals, measuring the grams of carbohydrate in them, and then giving a precalculated insulin dose to see if it is correct relative to the carbs you are eating. After doing this regularly for a few weeks you will find that you can look at a lump of food on your plate and know how many grams of carbohydrates it contains. Ultimately, carb counting gives you freedom in your diet that you couldn't have otherwise.

Other tools to count carbohydrates are right at hand (so to speak) and easy to use. For example, your thumb is about equal to a 1-ounce serving; a thumb tip is about a teaspoonful. Fist and palm sizes vary more, but generally a man's fist equals 3 to 4 servings in a man and a woman's equals 2 to 3 servings. This equates to 1 to 2 cups in volume. An average palm is equal to approximately 3 to 4 ounces, and a cupped handful equals 1 to 2 ounces. Using snack food as an example, a handful of nuts is 1 ounce; 2 ounces of pretzels are two handfuls. You may want to measure various foods relative to the size of your hand when you are home so you will know its exact equivalent measure. Then you'll be able to use it to estimate portion sizes when you are out. (See the table on page 110 for more examples of judging portion sizes using this method.)

Reading Labels: A Healthy Habit

The labels on prepared foods allow you to read the amount of carbohydrate in each serving. Knowing this can help you judge how much insulin to give. However, you must be sure you also know what is considered a serving size. You'll be surprised at how small a serving size can be, especially for calorie-dense foods like ice cream. More often than not, we end up eating more than one serving size. If you do you'll need to multiply the grams of carbohydrates by the number of serving sizes you are eating.

When my patients start carb counting, they tend to assume all carbs are equal. But over time they figure out that some carbs increase blood sugar levels more than others. What you should look at on food labels is the *total* amount of carbohydrate, rather than the separate types of carbohydrates listed, including sugar.

One other caveat regarding labels has to do with the many food products that call themselves "low fat." Often these foods are lower in fat than other alternatives, but they may contain excessive amounts of sugar or sodium to make up for compromised flavor. If you want an eye-opener, check the labels on those little containers of low-fat yogurt. Some may contain more than 20 or 30 grams of sugar. And although sugar is not the enemy, as I've said earlier, all this extra sugar doesn't help your blood sugar control—even with carb counting. Eating a lot of these low-fat but high-sugar or high-sodium products in the name of weight control is kind of like ordering a cheeseburger and fries with your diet soda.

New Carbohydrates

The food industry, in an effort to promote low-carbohydrate products, has been generating new terminology lately for describing carbohydrates. On many packages you now see "effective carbs," "net carbs," and/or "impact carbs" listed. This can be very confusing and sometimes misleading. These terms refer to fiber and sugar alcohols that the food industry claims have no effect on blood sugar levels. Unfortunately, this may affect your accuracy in determining your insulin to carbohydrate ratio. You should work with your nutritionist to learn how to account for sugar alcohol and fiber in your diet as it does not work the same for everyone.

Using the Glycemic Index

The glycemic index is a way of comparing one carbohydrate to another. Although we know that carbohydrate raises blood sugar levels, we also know (and as you probably know from experience) that some types of carbohydrate raise your blood sugar levels more than others. To develop the glycemic index, investigators gave people with type 1 diabetes a standard amount of sugar and measured how much it raised their blood sugar level after it was eaten. They gave this basic response an index level of 100. If the diabetics ate the same amount of a different carbohydrate and their blood sugar level didn't go up as high, it meant the new carb had a lower glycemic index. So, for example, they ate 15 grams of lentils their blood sugar went up only half as much as after eating 15 grams of white bread; therefore the glycemic index of lentils is

50. If the blood sugar response is greater, then the glycemic index is higher. Each of us will vary in terms of how we respond to carbohydrates, but this is a good general guideline for how much different carbs will raise your blood sugars.

Ideally, the food you eat would all be high in fiber and would have a lower glycemic index, because it would reduce your insulin requirements and make your diabetes easier to manage. Most of our diet, though, is made up of more processed foods, which have a higher glycemic index. Knowing a specific food item's glycemic index can be helpful. But an easier way to account for the glycemic index of foods is to know the carbohydrate and fiber content of each food you eat. If the dietary fiber listed on the label is 5 or more grams, you can subtract it from the total carbohydrate. Depending on the total grams of fiber of the meal, you would lower your insulin dose based on your carb to insulin ratio. I know this sounds difficult, but once you get the hang of it, it becomes second nature.

GETTING A HANDLE ON THE DIABETIC DIET

For many years we treated type 1 diabetes by prescribing strict diets, with fixed ratios of carbohydrate, fat, and protein. This was because we didn't have glucose meters until the mid 1980s, and people couldn't easily and accurately measure their premeal blood sugar levels and adjust their insulin doses. I don't think the concept of carbohydrate counting really caught on until we started having insulin analogues available for use, which increased our ability to mesh insulin and food intake. Most of the patients who come to see me still don't do much carbohydrate counting until we teach them. Newer, more flexible insulin regimens take a lot of time to teach and monitor, especially at first, and many patients haven't had access to a diabetes management team.

In the 1980s we were doing a lot of research to try to determine the best approach to the diabetic diet. Along with my mentor, Dr. Mayer Davidson, I did a research study called the Chocolate Cake Study that helped change how people with diabetes eat. In this study I continuously measured the blood sugars in people with a big machine called a Biostator, which worked like an artificial pancreas. I had people with type 1 diabetes sit in a big chair while I measured their blood sugar levels all day long. We studied the effect of adding and subtracting various foods in the diet. In the Chocolate Cake Study we had people eat two meals with an identical composition of carbs, fat, and protein—one day the meal included a baked potato and the next day we substituted a piece of chocolate cake for the potato. What we (and others) found was you could eat either a piece of cake or a baked potato in your meal—as long as you kept the carbohydrate content similar. Before this research we thought that people with diabetes had to avoid eating sugary desserts. In fact, some of my patients tell me sad stories of being a child with diabetes and either being shunned from birthday parties (because no one knew what to do) or being given an apple to eat while everyone else ate cake. After the study we were able to give much more flexible dietary advice and help people with diabetes live more normal lives.

BREAKING THE CARBOHYDRATE CODE

There are five basic types of carbohydrates: starches, fruits, vegetables, some dairy products (milk and yogurt), and simple sugars. Fiber is also a carbohydrate—with no calories—and some forms of alcohol (particularly when served as mixed drinks) count as carbohydrate, as well. When first learning carb counting, eating at home is less hassle than eating out. You can weigh and measure your food, compared to going out to a restaurant where you don't always know what things have been added to the food that could increase your blood sugar levels. Just do your best when you go out. Often you can ask for foods prepared simply, such as grilled without breading or a sauce, which will make carbohydrate counting easier.

Starches

Starches are long chains of sugar molecules and are often the hardest food content to measure accurately. I have had some patients tell me, "I am just not going to eat a baked potato. It makes my blood sugar level go up too high." Others find pasta or rice most difficult. Whatever your response to any given starch, it is important for you to be able to measure it. This starts by figuring out portion size. The basic portion size is ½ cup of *cooked* starch. Measure out half a cup of pasta or potatoes to see what it looks like. Most ½-cup servings are equal to 15 grams of carbohydrate, except for rice. Rice is extremely dense and ⅓ cup of white rice equals 15 grams.

Other starch servings that equal 15 grams of carbohydrate are 1 slice of bread or ½ cup of potatoes, garbanzo beans, kidney beans, lima beans, lentils, squashes, peas, croutons, or corn. Since many of these starches are added into salads or dishes in restaurants, it helps if you measure out 15 grams' worth at home to get a feel for what it will look like when mixed into your food when you eat out.

Fruits

Fruits are a good source of carbohydrate and are filled with lots of wonderful nutrients, minerals, and vitamins. Although the sugar in fruit can increase blood sugar levels, fresh fruit generally contains enough fiber to blunt some of the expected increase. Cooking fruit or mashing it to make fruit juice not only can increase the amount of carbohydrate consumed, it can lower the fiber content and increase the speed of the rise of blood sugar levels. I recommend trying to eat fresh fruit as often as you can. Really dense fruit like bananas are the exception. They can often raise your blood sugar levels too high. The portion size for a banana is half a banana—a whole banana is two portions (or equivalent to 30 grams of carbohydrate).

The difficulty in counting fruit carbs is that fruit doesn't come in premeasured sizes. Although sometimes fruit in the grocery store looks like it was made in a standard mold, natural fruit varies in size. It also varies in ripeness, which can alter its sweetness (or how much simple sugar is in the piece of fruit). In spite of this, it would be great if you could eat two to four servings of fruit per day. I personally don't come anywhere close to this—if I'm lucky I might eat three or four pieces of fruit per week. But I always feel like I'm doing something healthy for my body when I eat fruit, and I encourage you to do so.

In order to incorporate fruit into your diet, you need to follow these general rules: A very small apple, a small peach, or a small

pear equals 15 grams of carbohydrate. If you get huge ones from
the grocery store, you may need to count each as 20 to 25 grams. If
you eat a whole banana or grapefruit, it is worth 30 grams. If you
decide to drink fruit juice, which I generally don't recommend unless you are really fond of it (water is a better way to quench your
thirst, without the sugar calories), 4 ounces (or ½ cup) is 15 grams
of carbohydrate. It's a good idea to measure your drinking glasses
at home to determine how many ounces you are really drinking.

Vegetables

Vegetables are essential for a healthy diet. When you fill up your
plate with food, half the total amount should be vegetables. This
will provide you with essential nutrients and fiber, and will help
keep your weight in a good range. Vegetables are nutrient-dense.
This means that their store of nutrients is high compared to their
calorie content. Vegetables are easy to prepare and most can be
eaten either cooked or raw.

In the past, patients did not have to count nonstarchy vegetables when calculating carbohydrate grams. But now you do. They
are carbohydrates, after all, and healthy as they are, they can raise
your blood sugar. Therefore, consider 3 cups of nonstarchy *raw*
vegetables the equivalent of 15 grams of carbohydrate; and 1½ cups
of *cooked* vegetables (three times the portion size of one starch
serving) equal to 15 grams.

Dairy Products

Dairy products often contain carbohydrate, fat, and protein. They
also supply calcium, vitamin D, and other important vitamins and
minerals. It is best to consume low-fat dairy products to cut back
on your saturated fat and cholesterol consumption. Often when
you buy dairy products you can read on the container how many
grams of carbohydrate are in a serving. For milk, 8 ounces equals
12 to 15 grams of carbohydrate. Other skim milk products such
as buttermilk (8 ounces), hot cocoa (1 envelope of an artificially
sweetened mix), and yogurt (8 ounces nonfat, plain, or artificially
sweetened) can be included in a healthy diabetic diet.

Simple Sugars

Carbohydrates in the form of simple sugars increase your blood sugar levels quickly. We recommend that you consume 15 grams of simple carbohydrate to treat a low blood sugar reaction. Fifteen grams of sugar is equal to 2 tablespoons of table sugar, 1 tablespoon of honey, 4 ounces of juice, or 8 ounces of nonfat milk. Nondiet sodas contain a lot of simple sugar—approximately 8 teaspoons of sugar in a 12-ounce can. High-fructose corn syrups also are used in many foods and can raise blood sugar levels rapidly, usually in five to ten minutes. Even large amounts of catsup (which can be loaded with sugar) can increase your blood sugar levels. You need to be a detective, to find the hidden carbohydrate calories so you can adjust your insulin appropriately. On the food label you will find an ingredient list that tells you what type of sugar the food contains. If the word ends in *-ose*, it's sugar. Examples include: dextrose, fructose, maltose, lactose, and sucrose. The more you know, the better you'll function as a surrogate pancreas. And the better a pancreas you are, the more normal your blood sugar levels will be.

The more you know, the better you'll function as a surrogate pancreas.

Another approach is to log your food, its estimated carbohydrate content, and insulin doses given each day in order to get a sense of exactly what you are doing. Using your logs, I can see if your blood sugar levels before eating and two hours after are within range. If not, we can adjust your carbohydrate ratios and correction factors to make them more adequately cover your carbohydrate intake.

Fiber

Fiber is a form of carbohydrate that is indigestible, which means that it is not converted to sugar in the bloodstream. Fiber slows down the absorption of food, and in some studies has helped lower levels of glucose and fat absorbed into the blood after eating. However, this often requires that we eat large amounts of fiber, which can be hard to tolerate.

Overall, fiber is very good for us—it helps our system function normally. More fiber lowers the glycemic index of food and reduces how high the blood sugar levels go after we eat. The more we refine food, the more we break down fiber and the more readily the food is absorbed. When you count carbs, you will learn how fiber alters the absorption of the foods you commonly eat. If you read labels, or note in your carbohydrate counting book that the food you are eating contains 5 grams of fiber or more, you should subtract it from the carbohydrate total for that meal. For example, a breakfast cereal containing 23 grams of carbohydrate per serving with 13 grams of fiber can be counted as 10 grams of carbohydrate (23 minus 13).

Most Americans don't get enough fiber. It's recommended that adults eat 20 to 35 grams per day. Eating more fiber can aid weight loss and can help lower cholesterol levels. As you increase your fiber intake make sure you drink adequate amounts of fluid to avoid constipation.

Common sources of soluble fiber are oats and oatmeal; oat bran, rice bran, and corn bran; barley; dried peas; and kidney beans, pinto beans, and black beans. Sources of insoluble fiber include whole grains and whole grain products (cereal, pasta, bread, crackers); brown rice; raw vegetables; and fresh fruit.

Alcohol

Alcohol doesn't usually raise blood sugar levels by itself. In fact, pure alcohol reduces how much sugar your liver makes, and it can lower your blood sugar level. So we recommend that you always eat something when you drink, in order to avoid low blood sugar reactions. An alcoholic drink, however, doesn't always lower your blood sugar levels. Sometimes alcohol is combined with sweet mixers and juices and you need to take these into account. Examples include:

Strawberry daiquiri (12 ounces): 36 grams carbohydrate

Margarita (12 ounces): 48 grams carbohydrate

Piña colada (12 ounces): 48 grams carbohydrate

Fuzzy navel (12 ounces): 42 grams carbohydrate

Vodka martini (4 ounces): 40 grams carbohydrate

If you drink, you should learn the impact of various types of alcohol on your blood sugar levels. For example, beer has more carbs than wine.

From a health perspective, drinking a small amount of alcohol is probably good for you. Too much alcohol is clearly bad—brain and liver cells start dying—but a glass of wine with dinner may help lower your risk of heart disease. This has been studied in people both with and without diabetes. So although I don't tell people who don't drink to start drinking, I do tell people who drink in moderation that it's okay to continue. If you drink more than a little, you need to be concerned about low blood sugar reactions. I have patients who have to reduce or even withhold their overnight dose of insulin when they go out drinking. And although I don't advocate drinking to excess, if you do it is important to know how to anticipate the effect on your blood sugar levels so you can avoid serious low blood sugar reactions.

To count your alcohol calories and carbohydrates, follow these rules:

1. One drink is 12 ounces of beer, 5 ounces of wine, or 1½ ounces of distilled spirits.

2. If alcohol is used daily, the calories should be counted in the meal plan. If you are concerned about weight gain, alcohol is substituted for the fat serving. One drink of alcohol is considered to equal two fat servings.

3. Remember to take into account the calories and carbs of any mixers or juices used.

THE EFFECTS OF PROTEIN AND FAT ON BLOOD SUGAR LEVELS

Protein also converts into sugar, generally in a slow and gradual way. You don't really notice an increase in blood sugar levels after eating, say, 3 or 4 ounces of protein. However, if you eat 10 ounces of protein or more you will need to take extra insulin. When I did research studies on the effects of increasing protein in the diet, I found that it took four to six hours to see an increase in blood sugar levels when an additional 4 ounces of protein was added to the diet. This is a comparatively gradual increase in blood sugar levels. This showed that eating protein can help sustain blood sugar levels in the normal range, especially overnight or during other periods where there are long intervals between meals.

Fat slows gastric emptying and can prolong the effects of food in your system. Restaurant meals are larger and tend to have more protein and hidden fat, especially in Chinese and Mexican foods. Additionally, patients often tell me that eating pizza, which has both refined carbohydrate in the crust and lots of cheese (fat) in the topping, will cause their blood sugar levels to rise many hours later. If they want to eat pizza and are using an insulin pump, we can have them give their mealtime bolus over a long period of time, or give a small, second bolus dose of insulin an hour or two after the first, to smooth out the blood sugar rise. Fat itself never turns into sugar. Fats do add flavor and moisture to food, but have few vitamins and minerals. They are very caloric, with 9 calories per gram of fat. So serving sizes of all fats are small; choose monounsaturated fats over saturated or trans fats. See pages 105–108 for more discussion of dietary fats, as well as common food sources of the various types of fat.

GAINING FLEXIBILITY THROUGH CARB COUNTING

The first reason to learn carbohydrate counting is because it gives you more flexibility in terms of what and when you eat. It also helps you better mesh your insulin and blood sugar levels, helping you to avoid high and low blood sugar reactions. In terms of weight, however, I have seen people both gain and lose weight when they learn how to count carbs. The weight gain comes from the fact that once you can eat whatever you want, freed from the fear of high blood sugar levels, you might increase both your calories as well as your insulin dosing. Remember, insulin helps your body store calories, so more insulin plus more calories equals more fat. In general, if you want to lose weight you will want to cut back on calories, carbohydrates, and the insulin given. You don't want your blood sugar levels to become too high as a result. But in my experience knowing how to count carbs allows you to safely cut back on carbs and lose weight. Remember, though, that just as for people without diabetes, losing weight requires discipline and exercise, too.

One of the big positives to more flexible insulin regimens is that you no longer have to eat for your insulin. Insulins such as NPH and regular have a peak at a predictable time and you have to eat accordingly. If you don't eat, you end up with a low blood sugar reaction and then have to eat more than you would otherwise. I've had many patients lose weight when switching from a less flexible to a more flexible insulin regimen because suddenly they aren't a slave to eating for their insulin. They can control their calories and insulin instead of the other way around.

Carb Counting Made Simple

Carbohydrate counting is an important tool for you to use as you treat your diabetes. Although a bit tedious to learn, you won't be sorry that you spent the time to learn it. If you've had type 1 diabetes for a long time and were raised on the exchange system and the diabetic diet, you may be particularly resistant to changing. But what I've found is that people who have had diabetes for a while have learned a lot about carbohydrate counting through experience. Even if you're newly diabetic, it is fairly easy for you to guess that you are eating more carbohydrates when you eat a sweet dessert and that giving yourself extra insulin to cover it makes sense. The next step is to figure out how many grams of carbohydrates that dessert actually has and exactly how much insulin you need to cover the inevitable blood sugar rise. That's really all there is to carb counting. Once you are able to do it your eating patterns and lifestyle can become more flexible and, hopefully, somewhat less burdensome.

EIGHTEEN

THE EXERCISE ADVANTAGE

Patients with type 1 diabetes should exercise, just like people without diabetes. Exercise has many benefits (you already know this!) and I encourage everyone to do it, within the limits of their overall health. When you have type 1 diabetes and you exercise, certain adjustments need to be made. Exercise may change your insulin requirements, both before and after the activity. The story of my patient Brooke describes her challenges as she tried to compete as a woman with diabetes.

"A different way to measure myself."

Every fall. Harvest. A time to gather, I am gathering myself together. This is the time of year when one gathers strength and endurance for the winter that imposes itself on us . . . I am preparing. I am readying myself for an event. A race against myself called "Stair Climb to the Top." A big, boastful name. I tell no one. I am stretching my capabilities beyond reason. I am gathering courage to do this foolish thing again this year.

I do not know why I am terrorizing myself again. Why am I doing something so difficult? I need this justification to fill in a hole of incompleteness. Of feeling inadequate. Of not meeting some expectation or productivity level. It is proof, my proof, that I can defy my diabetes. I will outsmart it. I will challenge every blood sugar level that I come across. I need something to hold on to. I need something that can define me beyond illness. A different way to measure myself.

To get ready for the climb to the top I practice three to four times a week for several months. I find a set of weathered stairs cradled in a

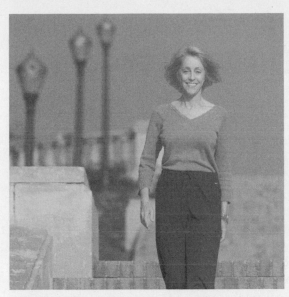

side of a mountain
in Santa Monica.
One hundred and
sixty-eight steps.
Eight stories. I need
to practice only go-
ing up but that is
not possible. The
stair climb is up
only. Seventy-five
flights. One thou-
sand five hundred
steps inside the
tallest building in
Los Angeles. The
Library Tower.

I sit in my car
gathering my energy to begin a practice round. I shove the seat back in
order to have enough room to change into my workout clothes. Lifting
my skirt discreetly, I squeeze into black stretch pants. I pull on my socks
and running shoes and tie the laces in a tight double bow so they will
not distract or cause a fall. I have a T-shirt hidden under my sweater.
I strap on my running watch. I test my blood, as I must always do before exercise, and slowly get out of my car. I am never in a hurry to
start. I carry a bottle of water, often warm from the long car ride. I
stretch for a few seconds to lessen the guilt of sore muscles afterward
and I begin the descent. I must look down at each step to keep my balance. I try to pick up the pace to get my heart rate moving. Soon I get
to the bottom. Without stopping, I turn around and start the trip back
up. Stopping would make it difficult to begin again. The climb up
cannot be done fast. One step at a time. One set at a time. How many
sets have I promised myself today? The first three sets are the most gru-
eling. All I can think about is how difficult it is. I try to count and
breathe. I focus on my breath. Nothing works. Can I meet my self-
imposed schedule?

The stairs never get easier. However, with each practice round I know
that I am closer to feeling a little better about myself. I do not always
feel well before, during, or after exercise. Exercise makes blood sugar

*control even more of a challenge. If there is not enough injected insulin
on board and the sugar level is high before exercising then the sugars
may be even higher after a workout. High sugars slow the system.
Muscles are not getting the necessary energy into their cells. The stair
climb then feels like torture. The body feels depleted. It is hard to tell if
the sugar is rising or falling during exercise. It is always a guess.
Every workout is a surprise. . . .*

*The night before the race I am extremely careful about what I eat.
More cautious than normal. I need to have energy. I awaken at three
AM with my heart pounding, a sure sign of low blood sugar. I pop two
glucose tablets into my mouth, put a pillow over my head, and try to
think of nothingness. Sleep does not arrive. All I can do is rest. I get up
at six AM and find my blood test to be 63. Way too low for exercise. I
feel horrible, tired, jittery, nauseated. I eat, inject insulin, shower, and
talk myself into feeling better because no matter what, I am going to do
the stair climb. I am frantically disappointed that I am not feeling well.*

*I drive to the race through fog and dim light, through the colorful
Korean and Hispanic sections of the city. I am ready to collapse. I am
angry that my body continues to let me down. An ugly little voice
inside me tells me that I am not capable, that I have no right to be
doing this with my erratic health. With great force I break away from
these thoughts and tell myself over and over that I can do this. I can do
this. I repeat these words until I reach the parking structure downtown.*

*I take another blood test. It reads 150. I am pleased. This is an
ideal number for exercise. I begin to relax a little about my blood sugar.
I chat with the other stair climbers. We are an odd-looking group. No
one looks particularly athletic. Anxiety is rising.*

*An announcement is made over the loudspeaker: "Fifteen minutes
to starting time." Time for one last blood test. One fifty-eight, still
good. My doctor suggested injecting two units of regular insulin just
prior to the race because as the adrenaline kicks in, the sugar rises.
I do not trust her system. I must make a quick decision since everyone
is lining up. I inject half a unit, stuff my sweatshirt and car keys into
a plastic storage bag, and get in line. The fog has lifted. Without
thinking I look up to the top and instantly my body fills with fear.
The building appears extraordinarily high. I cannot do this. I must
do this. I feel like I am about to be shot out of a cannon.*

The music starts up, our names are announced one at a time. I run

*through the balloon arch to the bottom of the stairwell. I begin the
ascent . . . I start a little too quickly. . . . Settle down. . . . Someone in
front of me is very slow . . . I speed up and then find I am breathing
too hard. . . . I pass three others and am feeling smug but know the
feeling is temporary.*

*I need to keep my pace to finish in a decent time. I try not to look at
the black numbers painted on the wall of each floor. I can't bear to see
that I'm only on the eighteenth floor when I'm already feeling drained
and doubtful. I look anyway—and often. At the twenty-fifth floor
I worry that I'm in trouble. Only a third of the way through and my
legs are beginning to tighten. I am grateful that I carry a water bottle.
I sip from it throughout the climb. As breathing becomes more difficult
I find the water a great comfort. I had passed five people but now
others are passing me. I step close to the handrail as others go by. . . .*

*The stairwell is disorienting and dusty. My mind is filled with
thoughts that evaporate just as they are being formed. I feel an
occasional sharp pain in my lungs. A day in the coal mines. The
stairwell takes a turn and throws off my pace. For sixty-six flights we
had been turning to the right; now we have to climb to the left. A big
adjustment. No choice. I try not to think about getting close to the
finish. I am determined not to look around to see how the others are
doing. I concentrate on taking one step at a time. It's a large task.
My mind and body are overloaded. I had planned to sprint to the top
but I have nothing left in me. I continue to the 72nd floor, then the
73rd. I hear loud music and great cheering. The 74th and finally the
75th floor. Yes! I've done it. I am outside, on the deck of the tallest
building in Los Angeles. In fresh air.*

*But I feel rotten. Something is wrong. I sit down, grab a towel,
and reach into my fanny pack to take out my blood meter, strips, and
lancet. My blood test results are 274. A normal person would test
between 70 and 110. Diabetes has interfered. The disease has gotten a
foothold and robbed me of feeling strong, healthy, and athletic. What a
huge disappointment! I do not have the ability to control glucose levels
even though I sometimes pretend I can. The high sugars make me feel
fatigued and nauseated. No wonder I am breathing so hard. My lungs
feel shredded. My head aches. I drink the rest of my water and inject
three units of insulin. I can't celebrate. Where's my moment of joy?
Simply finishing doesn't seem to matter, not right now anyway.*

I walk down a few flights and take the elevator to the 66th floor.
The victory floor. A group is gathering. We're waiting for the results to
be posted. I wrap my prize, a large loud T-shirt, around my sweaty body
and pace the cement floor while viewing the enormous city below. The
results finally come in. I have done the climb in twenty-three minutes,
not my personal best. Not at all what I had hoped for. I get into the ele-
vator and walk to my car in a glum mood. I drive home in silence.

Later, my daughter calls. "So, Mom, how did you do?"
"Not great," I say. "I wanted to be faster. If I didn't have diabetes
I would have done it so much better."

To which my wise daughter replies, "If you didn't have diabetes,
you probably would not have climbed the stairs at all."

She gathers me back together.

Whenever I drive east, toward downtown on a clear day in Los
Angeles, the Library Tower stands as a giant among the other buildings.
Every time I see that building I feel triumphant, knowing that for a
brief moment I conquered the fear of the stairs and the craziness of
diabetes. I have climbed to the top. I have completed the task.

....

Writing about exercise in patients with type 1 diabetes is one of
my very favorite topics. This is partly because I view it as a challenge. It is like working on a puzzle, meshing exercise, food, insulin, and stress and having it all come out right. And to know that
I can help my patients run marathons, compete in cross-country
races, and even win Olympic gold medals in swimming, makes it
exhilarating. My patient Brooke, in the story above, who has had
type 1 diabetes for thirty-five years, has three grown children, extraordinary control of her blood sugars, and no complications.
Part of her success is due to her commitment to exercise. It is part
of what keeps her healthy and thriving.

WHY EXERCISE?

Exercise for a person with type 1 diabetes has the same benefits it
does for the rest of us without diabetes. Exercise helps maintain
lean body mass and fight the effects of aging. It helps lower rates

of heart disease, cancer, obesity, and osteoporosis. It also gives a sense of well-being and helps us look better. Exercise increases strength and flexibility. It improves the fat levels in your bloodstream, lowering triglycerides and increasing the HDL (good) cholesterol in your blood. It helps fight stress and even improves sleep. Exercise also lowers insulin resistance (although people with type 1 diabetes often don't have a lot of insulin resistance and many are not overweight). I think that everyone needs to exercise five days a week for at least thirty minutes—ideally an hour—at a time.

Many people tell me how much they hate to exercise and they look at me as though I'm asking them to do something impossible when I tell them they should. The mistake people often make is that they think I am trying to give them a new leisure-time activity. I am not. I don't think there is anything fun about repetitive exercising for fitness. I consider exercise an assignment, a task you need to do to stay young, healthy, and fit. Most people don't mind participating in sports. But I know very few people who actually like the rote, boring, repetitive kind of exercise that is required to simply stay in shape.

Everyone needs to exercise five days a week for at least thirty minutes—ideally an hour—at a time.

I personally dislike exercise. Every second I am exercising I think about how soon I can stop. My brain is engaged in a continuous conflict between my desire to quit and my intellectual commitment to stay fit. Since it is always a struggle you'd think I'd give up. But do you know what I hate even more than exercising? Being out of shape. I hate how I feel if I don't exercise. And although I dislike the act of exercising, I am always glad I've done it.

I am definitely not a saint about exercise. There are weeks in which I can only exercise once or twice and there are occasional weeks when I go on strike because my body needs a break. But the following week I'm back to the routine. These are my own personal pointers for exercise that might help you.

1. Have a firm intellectual commitment to exercise—make it an ongoing priority.

2. Make a consistent time in your schedule that can be reliably free for exercise. I do it in the evening, from nine to ten PM, after my son is in bed and I have some time to myself.

3. Find a type of exercise that you can do comfortably. For me it's using a treadmill, an Exercycle, and a Bowflex machine. I can't go out at night and leave my son, so I have to have exercise equipment at home. We don't have a lot of space so we dedicated space in our living room to exercise.

4. Create a distraction to keep your mind off the exercise. I get nauseated if I read while I exercise, so I find a TV show to watch each night of the week.

5. Have reasonable expectations. Exercise will make you feel firmer, fitter, and more energetic. But you need to start slowly and build up gradually. And you may never like it. That doesn't matter; it's just something you need to do.

6. Drink plenty of fluids before, during, and after exercise. Being dehydrated can make blood sugar levels go up and you want to be sure that you drink enough water to prevent this.

ADJUSTING INSULIN FOR EXERCISE

When you exercise, your body becomes more sensitive to insulin. Therefore you will need to cut back on how much insulin you take before and after you exercise. Some people on insulin pumps will suspend their pumps during exercise, and turn the pump back on when they are done. This works well unless the exercise session lasts for more than an hour or is particularly intense. In that case, you will need some insulin again to keep your blood sugar levels from going up.

As with all things in diabetes, individualizing your treatment plan is the most important thing you can do. The amount you will need to change your insulin dose depends on how intense your exercise is. In addition to cutting back on your insulin dose, you may need to eat 15 to 30 grams of carbohydrate every thirty minutes during, and sometimes before exercising, to keep your blood sugar levels stable and in the normal range. Ideally, you won't have to eat lots of extra calories to keep your blood sugar level up. Still, active exercisers must always have some form of rapid-acting carbohydrate with them to treat a low reaction, if one should occur.

The best time to exercise is ninety minutes after eating. This is when the rapid-acting insulin is leaving your system and you have a good level of sugar in your blood. If you are going to be exercising strenuously, or if based on experience you know your blood sugar levels will fall too low, you may need to reduce the dose of insulin for the meal just before you exercise by 10 to 50 percent. You may also need to reduce the insulin dose prior to the next meal following exercise, as well. In addition, exercise during the day can lead to an increase in insulin sensitivity overnight. So some people need to decrease their dose of basal or long-acting insulin on the days they exercise, or eat a bedtime snack to prevent low blood sugar levels while they are sleeping.

If you are going to be exercising strenuously, or if based on experience you know your blood sugar levels will fall too low, you may need to reduce the dose of insulin for the meal just before you exercise by 10 to 50 percent.

The way I suggest learning your reaction to exercise is to test your blood sugar level just before and then right after you exercise. Keep track of what time you exercise and for how long, what you eat before, during, and after you exercise. This will help you develop a sense of your body's response to exercise. Some people have more than one insulin regimen for exercise. For example, they give themselves less insulin on the days when they do more cardiovascular work and more insulin on the days when they do primarily weight training.

Sometimes if your blood sugar is high before exercise, you may not want to exercise because strenuous activity can push it up higher. But in general, if it is high because of eating extra carbohydrate and you keep track of your blood sugars while you exercise (and drink plenty of fluids) you'll be okay. If it is high because you are getting sick, and your body is more insulin resistant due to illness, then you might not want to exercise that day or you might do a lighter workout. Again, the key to all of this is to test your blood sugar levels and learn your patterns. The best book on exercise and diabetes is _The Diabetic Athlete_ by Sheri Colberg. She has a PhD in exercise physiology and has type 1 diabetes herself, so she knows what she is talking about.

EXERCISE HAS ITS LIMITS

If you have no complications caused by diabetes you are free to exercise without restriction. However, if you are older than thirty-five you should ask your doctor before you begin an exercise program to be sure that you don't have any underlying heart disease. In some cases you will need to do a treadmill test to confirm that your heart is working fine before you begin an exercise program. If you have problems with your heart you may want to start your exercise in the setting of a supervised cardiac rehab program.

Diabetic eye disease or retinopathy can limit how much and what kind of exercise you should do. This is because the jarring of running or aerobics can put extra stress on the blood vessels in the back of your eyes and could cause them to burst and bleed. The same is true of lifting weights. You should be sure to have annual eye exams. If you have any diabetic eye damage you should ask your eye doctor (ophthalmologist) if it is okay to exercise.

Another limit to exercise can be diabetic nerve damage, particularly if your feet are involved or have ulcers on them. If you have loss of sensation in your feet you should be sure to see a podiatrist before you start exercising. That way, in addition to medical care, you can be fitted with special shoes that will protect your feet from any extra stress and strain that exercise might cause.

COMPETING WITH TYPE 1 DIABETES

When you do a mild to moderate workout, your blood sugar levels almost always fall. Your muscles are active and you are using glu-

cose for energy. But when you compete, or if you exercise strenuously, your body becomes stressed. When this happens you release
stress hormones, the catecholamines (epinephrine and norepinephrine), into your bloodstream. These hormones antagonize
the effect of insulin and make your blood sugar levels go up. This
is what happened to Brooke as she raced up the library building
stairs. I often have my athletic patients follow a different set of instructions for days when they are competing compared to days when
they are training. In order to compete effectively, athletes with diabetes need to be able to control blood sugar levels so their muscles get the necessary fuel to perform.

My favorite story about diabetes and sports is that of Gary Hall Jr.

More than any other area of managing diabetes, learning how
to handle exercise and competition is an art—an art of the possible.
The newer insulins and better, faster glucose meters increase the
management options. I rarely find a situation that I can't help fix
as long as patients are willing to test and learn from experience.

My favorite story about diabetes and sports is that of Gary Hall Jr.
When he discovered he had type 1 diabetes he was already an elite
athlete. He had won two gold and two silver medals in swimming
at the 1996 Atlanta Olympics and was training for the 2000 Sydney
Olympics. After his diagnosis, his local endocrinologist told him
that he had to give up competitive swimming. This was probably
because in world-class competition the difference between winning and losing a race often is measured in hundredths of a second. The physician Gary saw probably thought that it would be
impossible for someone with type 1 diabetes to optimize fuel
metabolism to achieve peak performance. But this doctor didn't
know Gary.

Through Gary's father, a physician, Gary found me and flew
from Phoenix to Los Angeles. Although at that point I knew a lot
about treating type 1 diabetes, I didn't know much about athletes
and type 1 diabetes. However, I was so impressed by Gary and his
interest in helping other people with diabetes that I gave him the

green light to try to continue competing. I didn't say I was sure it would work; but I thought it was worth finding out.

I flew up to Berkeley, where Gary was training, to sit by the side of the pool and measure his blood sugar levels. I needed to learn about competitive swimming and how to fashion an insulin regimen around his workouts and swim meets. I met his coach and worked with both of them on how to optimize Gary's nutrition. At first I was worried that Gary's blood sugar levels would fall too low in the pool and that he would be at risk for losing consciousness and drowning. But Gary was so in tune with his body and so diligent about testing that this proved not to be a problem. A bigger problem was that if he exercised too hard during the day he would become too low at night and we had to account for this.

I also went with Gary to his swim meets and learned how much the stress of competing could raise his blood sugar levels. Swimming only 50 meters could raise Gary's blood sugar level from 150 to 300 mg/dl during major competition, but swimming 100 meters during training would lower his blood sugar level from 150 to 90. I gained a lot from Gary as I watched him learn about his body and how it responded with diabetes. He was particularly diligent when it came to learning about nutrition and his diabetes—something that everyone needs to know.

In the end Gary's hard work paid off. I was with him at the Sydney Olympics where he won two gold medals, one silver, and one bronze. He had been all but written off before the Olympic Trials but came back to show the world what he could do, diabetes and all. The same thing happened when I was with him in Athens, where he shocked everyone by winning the gold medal in the 50-meter freestyle race. He won in spite of being older (nearly thirty) and having diabetes. A truly remarkable feat. Gary has learned to make diabetes a part of his life, as opposed to something that ruled his life.

....

"I realized I had a chance to encourage millions of people living and suffering with diabetes."

Now I've told my side of Gary's story. Here it is from his perspective. He wrote this while he was training for the Sydney Olympics.

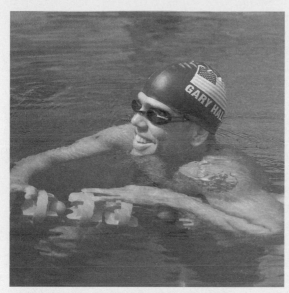

I was diagnosed with diabetes. My first reaction was a desire to fall down, even though I was sitting. I couldn't believe it. I thought that diabetes was a disease that happened to old people who had neglected their health for years, more years than I had been alive. I let out a sigh of defeat. I was filled with a hopeless void, and all I could do was just sit there in disbelief. I was upset. Upset like mad. Upset like disturbed. Upset in every sense of the word. I was furious. I was depressed, dumbfounded, and horrified. I was really scared.

I was a blank on the outside, asking the doctor, "What does this mean?" He said something about the good news being there have been tremendous steps taken in the past twenty years in treating the disease. The bad news was that I needed medication. Daily. By injection. Or I would die.

So I was sent to an endocrinologist. It was there that I was informed that my swimming career was over, at least as I knew it. I was desperate. Exasperated. I wanted to lunge at the doctor. I wanted to defy him. I wanted to defy the disease. But didn't know if I could. I had no idea what I was up against. I decided that I needed a vacation.

The endocrinologist actually called my grandmother, as well as my parents, to keep me from going to Costa Rica. But I went anyway. I packed up my insulin, my needles, my girlfriend, and my dog and headed south. I gathered as much information as I could before leaving. It was in Costa Rica that I did a lot of reading, and it was there that I began to have a better understanding of what diabetes was all about. I often felt self-destructive. I would do things like swim in *shark-infested waters, hoping for the worst. More than once the sharks would bump me from the break of a wave. But then I would return to my bungalow and learn more about diabetes.*

At first, all I could read were the horror stories of people who had lost their sight, lost their legs, lost their kidneys to diabetes. "But other than that," they'd say, "everything else is fine." And that was from the motivational section! As time passed, I came to terms with my disease. I knew that I must accept the circumstances and deal with it. I had no choice. Accept the cards you're dealt, or fold. I had been through so much in the past, had overcome so many obstacles. This was just another to be hurdled.

I returned from Costa Rica with a sense of peace. I immediately sought out a new doctor and was lucky to find the best, Dr. Anne Peters [then] out of UCLA. I met with her and discussed the possibilities. She was so encouraging. First of all, I had to fly in to see her. I was an hour late (flight delay) and she had an appointment on the other side of town. So she told me to come with her. How many doctors would do that? I spent the afternoon with her driving around Santa Monica in her VW bug talking about what should and could be done.

I was going to give swimming a try. I called my coach Mike Bottom, who was up in Berkeley, California. I told him that I wasn't sure if it was going to work. Many times it didn't work. Practice was constantly interrupted with blood tests. Dr. Peters flew up to Berkeley to monitor and observe. The training went on for a couple of months; in swimming this is considered a very short season. Five months after being diagnosed with diabetes, I won nationals. Not only did I win, but I dropped 0.13 of a second, which was the difference between the gold and silver medal in the Atlanta Olympics. So to me 0.13 of a second is a huge deal.

It was at this point in my career and life that I understood the opportunity that had presented itself. I realized I had a chance to encourage millions of people living and suffering with diabetes. What I had done, and what I could do, might offer hope to people of all ages who had experienced that awful diagnosis and the pain that follows, a hope that could somehow alleviate the feelings of helplessness and defeat. If I am able to do that, for just one person, it would be so much more of an accomplishment than anything I achieve in the pool.

I think Gary is a great inspiration to everyone with diabetes—and anyone else—because he proves that you can keep striving for your dreams. Although most of us don't aspire to win Olympic medals, every person with diabetes faces his or her own exercise-related challenges, whether it is climbing a tower of stairs or simply finding a way to work out every day. If you pay attention to your diabetes, develop a partnership with a knowledgeable health care team, and stick with it, exercise can greatly enhance the quality of your life. Who knows, you may decide to run a marathon after all.

A PRESCRIPTION FOR THE FUTURE

Diabetes can now be tamed but it cannot be cured. Someday, I know a cure will be found, although the cures for type 1 and type 2 diabetes are likely to be different and may involve multiple components. With every news bulletin of some "diabetes miracle drug" I am besieged with phone calls from hopeful patients. Little bits of research, an idea here or there, pieces of the puzzle, are adding up. I hope that soon someone may make a leap, like the one that led to the discovery of penicillin from bread mold. But exactly when and how that will happen I can't say. The only certainty is that when the answer comes, there will be years of testing required before it is safely translated to a product for widespread use in humans. Until that time, we need to accept each small advance in treatments and technology and combine them to keep advancing, extending what we can do to treat diabetes.

Think of Gary Hall Jr. He is a testament to what can be done when you have diabetes. He took the tools we have available now for the treatment of diabetes, and used them to pursue his Olympic dream. He learned by reading and learning and being aware of what existed and how it could help him succeed. He sought answers. And he didn't give up. The same determination infuses all the patients' stories shared in this book. It can be your story, too. Living well with diabetes, *in spite of* diabetes, requires a questioning mind and a willingness to explore for yourself what works and what doesn't. Diabetes is a disease where we have adequate, functional tools for success—as long as you are willing to use them.

I know that it is hard not to get your hopes up when you hear about some promising new treatment, only to find that it may be years and years before it becomes available—if it ever does. I get discouraged, too. But then I step back and take stock of all of the advances I have already seen since I came out of medical school. When I first started training as a doctor, the drugs we had were much, much more limited. We didn't have home blood sugar monitoring— people still had to rely on urine testing, which is pathetic and inaccurate by comparison. We had just started using A1C levels to determine the overall level of blood sugar control. And equally important, when I started training we didn't have firm data that showed how much good blood sugar control matters. That data came in the 1990s when we finally had irrefutably solid evidence that in both type 1 and type 2 diabetes blood sugar control was really crucial, even though prior to that we all suspected it was.

It was not until I had completed my training that the first of the statins, powerful cholesterol-lowering drugs, were released onto the market. At about the same time the ACE inhibitors, drugs for high blood pressure and kidney disease, were introduced. Finally, since the mid 1990s we have had an explosion of new oral antidiabetes drugs and insulin analogues. Now I'm confident that I can effectively treat every patient I see.

Frankly, I'd love to go out of business.

So when I look at the treatment of diabetes from a historical perspective, I am overwhelmed by how far we have come. And yet I can't help dreaming, of being impatient for better solutions. I dream of safely curing my insulin-requiring patients, of helping them live without needles and lancets and the ups and downs of insulin use. I pray for a drug that can help safely help reduce central fat, melting away high blood sugar and cholesterol levels. I dream of a foolproof way for preventing heart attacks and strokes. Frankly, I'd love to go out of business.

But until I am declared obsolete I remain dedicated to taking what we know and helping translate that information into healing patients and preventing complications of the disease. We know enough now to make life for those with diabetes much, much better. There is more hope than ever before in the field of diabetes research and I know that the future will only get brighter. So take the resources and tools that I have presented in these pages and learn how to help yourself. You can do it! Don't wait for the "cure" or the next miracle drug. Don't stop with reading this book. Always keep informed, learn about what is new out there, what may help you or your children someday. Keep asking questions and don't stop until you find answers that work for you. Remember that right now, even without all the answers, we have many tools for reducing the deadly toll of prediabetes and diabetes types 1 and 2. Yet far less than half of the people in America who need treatment are getting it. Be sure you not only are in the group that receives good care from a health care team, but that you provide your own good care by reaching and maintaining your targets for glucose, cholesterol, and blood pressure.

So never give up. Believe in yourself and in your power to find health care that heals. Each one of you with diabetes can do this. Your life literally depends on it.

DR. PETERS' PRESCRIPTION FOR HEALTHY LIVING WITH PREDIABETES AND DIABETES

1. Establish a Partnership

Find a health care team that answers your questions and encourages you to be a partner in your own treatment. Ideally this team will consist of a physician skilled in the prevention and treatment of diabetes, a nurse educator who is a certified diabetes educator (CDE), and a nutritionist. There are other health care providers who may also need to be part of your team, such as an ophthalmologist and a podiatrist, as needed.

2. Discover Your Family History

Uncover your family health history and be sure that relatives are screened early and regularly for prediabetes and heart disease. Almost everyone I see with prediabetes or type 2 diabetes has a family history of diabetes or heart disease. Knowing your family history helps determine your risk for having a similar health problem. This is equally important when it comes to other diseases—knowing you have a family history of colon or breast cancer, for example, should lead you to earlier screening and help to pick up early cancers before they spread.

3. Track Your Numbers

Know your numbers (glucose, lipids, blood pressure, kidney function), what they mean, and if you are on target (and if not, why not). Often physicians do not have complete flow sheets of your blood tests. You can easily keep track of your important laboratory values. You should track your kidney function, your cholesterol and triglycerides, your glucose levels and A1C values. If you keep following them over time, you can tell if a value is increasing or decreasing and can ask your doctor what it means. Sometimes it is hard to keep track of small changes in laboratory values, but as a patient you can monitor what is happening and ask to understand why.

4. Keep Records

Obtain a copy of all of your test results and bring it to your first appointment with any new provider. It really helps me when a patient brings in all of the tests from their past physician so I can look at what has been done before. You should keep a folder filled with all of your medical records. These records should be in chronological order—starting with the date furthest in the past and tracking up toward the present. You can let a new physician review your old records, and make a copy of them if needed, but don't give away your original copies. These reports represent your own personal health history and it is very important to provide this information to everyone who takes care of you in the future.

5. List Your Medications

Keep an updated list of your medications with you at all times. You may want to bring all of your pill bottles in with you to your doctor's appointments. I often find that patients bring in nicely typed lists that sometimes are incorrect; when I review the pills a patient is actually taking, it often doesn't match the list. As a physician, it is crucial for me to know all of the medications you are taking so I don't add any medication that doesn't mix well with the pills you are taking, or so I know what to change if a condition needs improving. If you didn't bring in your pills and you can't exactly remember what they are, there are pictures of many medications in the *Physician's Desk Reference* (*PDR*), a reference book found in many doctors' offices. You can often find the exact pills you are taking in this book, and pointing to pictures is often the most accurate way to remember your medications.

6. Eat Wisely

Work with a nutritionist to develop an individualized healthy-eating plan that you can stick with for life. This may seem difficult at first, but a good nutritionist will work with you to find an eating plan that fits with your lifestyle. Often, if you are overweight, small changes over time can result in weight loss and improvements in health. However, this is tough to do alone, and having either an individual (and nonjudgmental) nutritionist or being part of a group can help you make changes that last a lifetime.

7. Exercise Daily

Find a way to incorporate exercise (both aerobic and gentle weight training) into your life, at least five days a week, every week. Start slowly if you haven't been active, then gradually increase to a higher exercise intensity. If you are over thirty-five years old, your doctor may need to check out your heart before you start an exercise program to be sure it is safe. Someone on your diabetes team, whether it is the doctor, nurse educator, or nutritionist, should be able to work with you on your exercise program and make suggestions about what to do. To make yourself feel better, remember that all exercise counts. So if you are a mother racing around after small children or you walk a lot on the job, that helps your body stay healthy, too. You can get a pedometer to wear throughout the day, which will measure how many steps you are taking each day. This way, you can track your progress as you become healthier and also give yourself credit for some of the exercise you do when you aren't formally exercising. Don't be too tough on yourself if you miss a day or even a week. Just don't do it too often.

8. Test Sugars

Check your own blood sugar levels before and one or two hours after eating; learn what the numbers mean and what you should do about them. One of the few convenient things about diabetes is that it is numeric—you can test your blood sugar numbers on your own to determine if your medication and diet are working. You need to know what normal blood sugars are and what your own targets are, but you have the power to monitor yourself—what you eat, how you exercise, and when you take medication. You don't even need a prescription to buy a glucose meter, although if you have a prescription your insurance usually will pay for it. Having the ability to test takes away a lot of the guesswork and helps you understand what is happening in your body at a specific moment.

9. Know Side Effects

Ask about possible side effects for any new medications and what you can do to lower your risk of experiencing them. You must always remember that all drugs have benefits and risks. At the worst, all drugs can kill you, even ones you take without thinking, such as Tylenol or aspirin. Herbal preparations and vitamins are drugs, too. All have their own set of risks and benefits so you need to know what is in them and what they can do. On the plus side, medications can make a huge difference in your life. When I give someone a new drug I make sure the patient understands not only what the drug is doing (for instance, lowering blood sugar or cholesterol levels), but why the action is so important. Then I explain the common side effects, what to watch for, such as a cough or muscle pain or a stomachache. I also talk about the rare side effects, the ways in which the drug could cause serious problems, and try to help people learn how to avoid them. You can also look up side effects on the Internet or ask your pharmacist, but what you may get is a laundry list of possible problems and it may be hard for you to determine which ones are important to worry about and which ones aren't. You also need to have a sense of balance when reading about side effects. Remember, we prescribe drugs because we think their benefits are much greater than their risks. But you need to feel free to ask questions, to understand the medications that are prescribed for you, and to feel comfortable talking with your physician if you think you are having a reaction to the drug you are taking.

10. Monitor Drugs

Learn if special monitoring (for example, of liver, kidney, or red blood cells) is needed for any medication you are taking, and be sure to follow the recommendations. I am always surprised at how few patients know that there are strict guidelines for monitoring certain drugs and guidelines for when drugs should and shouldn't be used. I am equally surprised that often this monitoring isn't done by the doctors who prescribe the drugs. In general these rules are designed to protect you, the patient, and should be followed. It may mean coming into the doctor's office more often, but it is worth it. Many medications now have a "patient package insert" that will tell you the common side effects and need for monitoring. Be sure to read this insert and follow its instructions.

11. Stay Knowledgeable

Read everything you can, from books to newspapers, magazines to Internet posts, and make sure that your treatment is as current as possible. Medicine is always changing and all of us need to work hard to keep track of the changes. Often it is overwhelming. The media love to pick up on new "cures" that turn out to only work in odd strains of genetically altered mice. Such advances can have very little to do with treatments for actual humans. On the other hand, some new therapies are important and may impact the way you take care of your health. There are two issues that arise with new treatments. The first is that when a new drug comes on the market it has been tested in only a few thousand people and sometimes side effects don't show up until the drug has been used in tens of thousands of people. So new drugs carry unknown risks and you need to determine whether the benefits outweigh any potentially undiscovered risk. The second issue is that new drugs are always much more expensive than older drugs, and health plans may not want to pay for newer medications at first. So you should talk with your physician or someone in your health care team about new developments that interest you, and ask if they could help you. Then, perhaps call your insurance company and see if the new treatment is covered. The more you are informed, the more you go to local diabetes seminars, read diabetes magazines and books, and keep up-to-date, the better your health care will be.

12. Be Forgiving

Never expect perfection. Even if you have some bad days or even some bad months, you can always get back on track and take care of your health. None of us is perfect and that is particularly true when it comes to treating diabetes, which is a disease that involves making abrupt lifestyle changes as well as managing medications. There will be times when you don't feel like exercising or sticking to your meal plan. There may be times when you just can't poke your finger to measure your blood sugar like your doctor wants you to. You may really struggle with your weight and try your hardest and not see much change on the scale. All of this is okay. What matters is that you are trying to be healthier. Even if there are times when you find it impossible to do all of the things asked of you, don't despair. The key is to get back on track as soon as you can—if you have a bad day or two don't throw in the towel and stretch it out to a bad month or two. You just have to do the best you can. And that is the point with diabetes—one bad week won't cause irreparable harm, but a bad year or two can. So give yourself "diabetes holidays" if you need them (although be sure to keep taking your medications, especially your insulin if you are on it). None of us is perfect. All we can do is try. And with diabetes if you keep trying, you will be much, much healthier and happier than if you don't.

APPENDIX

SIMPLE MEAL OPTIONS

These are sample meals and snacks to give you ideas on how to create simple meal options. All meal suggestions can be interchanged with other types of carbohydrate, protein, and fat sources. You can also come up with other menu ideas by looking through your favorite magazines or cookbooks. You may need to modify the recipe by reducing the serving size, fat, or sodium to meet your nutritional needs. Remember this is not a diet, but a lifestyle change.

After you get some new menu ideas, take some time to plan out meals for the week. You may want to consider what you already have in your pantry and the season. Buying seasonal food always tastes better and is usually less expensive. Don't forget to add new flavor and textures to your meals through different herbs, marinades, and grated vegetables. When meals are planned ahead of time, you're more likely to be successful with your blood sugar control and weight management. Plus, it will reduce your stress and you will have more time to enjoy other activities with family and friends.

Ten Health Concepts for Life

1. Eat a minimum of two fruits and three vegetables daily.
   Try different colors of fruits and vegetables, which provide many disease-preventing nutrients like folic acid, vitamin C, fiber, and antioxidants, to name a few.

2. Count fiber grams; eat 25 to 30 grams of fiber each day.

3. Use fat in moderation. Choose plant sources (olive and canola oil, peanuts, almonds, walnuts, and avocados) over animal fats.

4. Limit processed foods (chips, crackers, cakes, and cookies). Sticking to fresh forms of food gives you more nutritional value and less sodium and trans-fatty acids.

5. Don't skip breakfast—eat small, frequent, and balanced meals throughout the day (three small meals and two snacks). Snacks should be less than 150 calories each.

6. Don't splurge when dining out. Skip the "free food," i.e., bread, chips, etc.

7. Drink lots of water.

8. Move your body daily.

9. Maintain a healthy body weight.

10. Most important: Be consistent! You will see the results if you give yourself time.

BREAKFAST OPTIONS

Berry Parfait

Blueberries/blackberries—
½ cup
Light yogurt—8 ounces
Almonds or walnuts—
5 chopped
Calories: 192 / Carbs: 30 grams

Almond and Jelly Delight

Whole wheat English muffin—1
Almond butter—1 tablespoon
Low-sugar fruit spread—
1 tablespoon
Calories: 263 / Carbs: 29 grams

Egg McMuffin

Whole wheat English muffin—½
Poached egg—1 (extra large)
Canadian bacon—1 ounce
Light margarine—1 teaspoon
Calories: 300 / Carbs: 27 grams

Breakfast Burrito

Whole wheat tortilla—8 inches
Pam butter spray
Egg Beaters scrambled—¼ cup
Add onions, peppers, and salsa
Low-fat shredded cheese—
1 ounce
Calories: 235 / Carbs: 25 grams

Egg White Veggie Scramble

Pam butter spray
Sauté onions, mushrooms, and
spinach
Add 3 egg whites
Whole wheat toast—1 slice
Light margarine—1 teaspoon
Strawberries—1 cup
Calories: 173 / Carbs: 30 grams

Pita Cheese Danish

Mini whole wheat pita—
2 ounces
Mix: low-fat ricotta cheese
(2 ounces), vanilla extract
(few drops), cinnamon and
sweetener to taste. *Broil until
cheese is melted.*
Raspberries—½ cup
Calories: 140 / Carbs: 22 grams

Crispy Waffle with Berries

Frozen Eggo Nutri-Grain
waffle—1
Light syrup—2 tablespoons
Blueberries—½ cup
Low-fat cottage cheese—
4 ounces
Calories: 215 / Carbs: 24 grams

Cheese Toasted Pita and Tomatoes

Whole wheat pita toasted—
  ½ (1 ounce)
Goat cheese (chèvre)—
  3 tablespoons (1 ounce)
Chopped tomatoes—⅓ cup
Pear—medium (6 ounces)
Calories: 225 / Carbs: 37 grams

Buckwheat Pancakes and Berries

Buckwheat pancakes—two-inch
Light margarine—2 teaspoons
Light syrup—2 tablespoons
Healthy Choice breakfast
  sausage—2 patties
Strawberries—6 medium or
  3 large
Calories: 220 / Carbs: 25 grams

Mango Salsa Quesadilla

Corn tortilla—one 6-inch
Shredded cheese—1 ounce
Trader Joe's mango salsa—
  2 tablespoons
Calories: 185 / Carbs: 23 grams

Cinnamon Oatmeal

Oatmeal—1 cup cooked
Cinnamon—½ teaspoon
Raisins—10
Nonfat milk—2 ounces
Calories: 187 / Carbs: 39 grams

Italian Vegetable Omelet

Egg Beaters—½ cup
Pam butter spray
Fresh basil—to taste
Chopped tomatoes—⅓ cup
Onions—2 tablespoons
Whole wheat roll—1 ounce
  (toasted with 1 teaspoon
  light margarine, garlic
  powder, 1 teaspoon
  Parmesan cheese)
Kiwi—medium (3 ounces)
Calories: 197 / Carbs: 25 grams

PB & J

Oroweat whole wheat bread—
  1 slice
Natural peanut butter—
  1 tablespoon
Low-sugar fruit spread—
  2 teaspoons
Apple (sliced)—1 small
  (4 ounces)
Calories: 281 / Carbs: 35 grams

High-Fiber Cereal and Yogurt

Kellogg's All-Bran cereal—
  ½ cup
Light yogurt—8 ounces
Raspberries—½ cup (fresh or
  frozen)
Calories: 220 / Carbs: 36 grams

LUNCH OPTIONS

Chicken Curry Salad

Chicken chunks—4 ounces
Apple (chopped)—⅓ cup
Low-fat plain yogurt—
  2 tablespoons
Curry powder—to taste
Mix above ingredients; place on a
  bed of salad greens.
Naan bread—¼ (8 by 2 inches)
Calories: 287 / Carbs: 28 grams

Middle Eastern Pita Pocket

Whole wheat pita—½
Hummus—2 tablespoons
Cucumbers (chopped)—¼ cup
Cherry tomatoes (chopped)—4
Lettuce (chopped)—¼ cup
Put above ingredients into pita
  pocket.
Side of tabouli—½ cup
Calories: 302 / Carbs: 24 grams

Vegetarian Sandwich

Whole wheat baguette—
  6 inches
Roasted peppers, onions,
  mushrooms, and eggplant—
  2 slices each
Fresh mozzarella cheese—
  1½ ounces
Trader Joe's pesto sauce—
  2 teaspoons
Calories: 350 / Carbs: 30 grams

Salad and Sandwich Combo

Tuna with nonfat mayo—
  2 ounces
Alpine Lace Swiss cheese—
  1 ounce
Lettuce and tomato
Rye bread—1 slice
Compile above ingredients into ½
  sandwich.
Mixed green salad—3 cups
Bernstein's light salad
  dressing—2 tablespoons
Calories: 310 / Carbs: 27 grams

Soup and Sandwich Combo

Smoked turkey—3 ounces
Sprouts and tomatoes
Mustard—1 tablespoon
Whole wheat bread—1 slice
Compile the above ingredients into
  ½ sandwich.
Pritikin vegetable soup—1 cup
Calories: 330 / Carbs: 39 grams

Sushi Plate

Miso soup—1 cup
Edamame (soybeans)—½ cup
Sushi—4 pieces
Sashimi—4 ounces (4 pieces)
Light soy sauce
Calories: 471 / Carbs: 33 grams

Open-Faced Italian Chicken Sandwich

Grilled chicken breast—
  3 ounces
Red sauce—2 tablespoons
Low-fat mozzarella cheese—
  ½ ounce
Focaccia bread—1 ounce
*Compile the above ingredients into
  open-faced sandwich.*
Mixed green salad
Low-calorie Italian dressing—
  2 tablespoons
Calories: 335 / Carbs: 31 grams

Cottage Cheese and Fruit Plate

Low-fat cottage cheese—1 cup
Strawberries—1 cup
Peach—½ medium
Calories: 240 / Carbs: 24 grams

BBQ Chicken Salad

BBQ chicken (skinless)—
  3 ounces
BBQ sauce—2 tablespoons
Romaine lettuce—3 cups
Corn—¼ cup
Tomatoes—1 small
Frito Lay baked corn chips
  (chopped)—3
Trader Joe's cilantro salad
  dressing (reduced fat)—
  2 tablespoons
Calories: 319 / Carbs: 24 grams

Mexican Beef Soft Taco

Corn tortillas—two 6-inch
Lean beef—3 ounces
Salsa, lettuce, and tomatoes
Light sour cream—1
  tablespoon (optional)
*Compile the above ingredients into
  2 tacos.*
Black beans—½ cup
*Calories: 357 to 382 /
Carbs: 39 grams*

Veggie Pizza and Salad

Veggie pizza (thin crust)—
  2 slices (6 ounces)
Mixed green salad—large
Light dressing—2 tablespoons
Calories: 355 / Carbs: 50 grams

Ham and Cheese Wrap

Whole wheat tortilla—one
  8-inch
Lean ham—2 ounces
Alpine Lace Swiss cheese—
  1 ounce
Lettuce and tomatoes
Hot'n'Sweet mustard—
  1 tablespoon
Calories: 375 / Carbs: 24 grams

Veggie Burger

Boca Original burger—one
  2½-ounce

Whole wheat bun—1½ ounce
Lettuce, red onions, tomatoes
Avocado—½ ounce
Light mayo—2 teaspoons
Mixed berries—1 cup
Calories: 300 / Carbs: 39 grams

Thai Stir-Fry

Mixed vegetables—3 cups
Thai peanut sauce—¼ cup
Chicken (skinless)—3 ounces
Cooked brown rice—½ cup
Calories: 390 / Carbs: 37 grams

DINNER OPTIONS

Wild Dill Salmon

Grilled wild salmon—4 ounces
Trader Joe's lemon dill sauce—
   2 tablespoons
Brown rice—½ cup
Asparagus—12 spears
Mixed green salad
Light dressing—2 tablespoons
Calories: 445 / Carbs: 32 grams

Roasted Chicken and
Sweet Potatoes

Roasted chicken—3 ounces
Sweet potatoes—1 medium
   (4 ounces)
Smart Balance light
   margarine—1 tablespoon
Cooked spinach—1 cup

Mixed green salad
Light salad dressing—
   2 tablespoons
Calories: 380 / Carbs: 36 grams

Vegetable Curry

Mixed vegetables—2 cups
Chickpeas—½ cup
TJ's Vegetable Curry Sauce—
   ¼ cup
Basmati rice (cooked)—½ cup
Green salad
Kraft Cucumber Ranch
   dressing—2 tablespoons
Calories: 437 / Carbs: 43 grams

Beef Fajitas

Grilled lean meat—3 ounces
Red, green peppers, and
   onions *sautéed* in 1 teaspoon
   canola oil
Salsa—½ cup
Corn tortillas   two 6 inch
Black beans—½ cup
Calories: 459 / Carbs: 41 grams

Roasted Pork

Roast lean pork tenderloin—
   4 ounces
String beans—1 cup
Butternut squash—1 cup
Light margarine—
   1 tablespoon
Mixed fruit—1 cup
Calories: 429 / Carbs: 43 grams

Shrimp Pasta Primavera

Shrimp—12 medium
Healthy Choice Vegetable
    Primavera—1 cup
Fettuccine noodles (cooked)—
    1 cup
Green salad
Bernstein's Light Roasted
    Garlic Balsamic dressing—
    2 tablespoons
Calories: 400 / Carbs: 41 grams

Chicken Marsala

Trader Joe's marsala sauce—
    ½ cup
Add extra mushrooms—½ cup
Chicken breast—3 ounces
Steamed zucchini—1 cup
Roasted red potatoes—
    3 ounces
Green salad
Girard's Lite Champagne
    dressing—2 tablespoons
Calories: 441 / Carbs: 43 grams

Stir-Fry Vegetables with Tofu

Tofu—6 ounces (cubed)
Mixed vegetables—4 cups
    (bok choy, mushrooms,
    onions, bean sprouts,
    broccoli, carrots)
*Combine the remaining ingredients
    into a sauce:*
Teriyaki sauce—2 tablespoons

Light soy sauce—1 tablespoon
Fresh garlic—to taste
Canola—2 teaspoons
Calories: 420 / Carbs: 35 grams

Amy's Organic Chili

Amy's Organic Chili—2 cups
    (has 7 grams fiber per cup)
Green onions (optional)
Chopped tomatoes (optional)
Fresh cilantro (optional)
Nonfat sour cream—
    1 tablespoon
*Heat chili and top with above
    ingredients.*
Spinach salad
Girard's Lite Champagne
    dressing—2 tablespoons
*Calories: 440 / Carbs: 38 (52
grams listed, minus 14 grams of fiber)*

Grilled Tuna Niçoise

Tuna, sliced—4 ounces
Marinate tuna in Girard's Lite
    Champagne dressing
    (3 tablespoons), *then grill.*
Red potatoes—3 ounces, grilled
Asparagus—6 spears, grilled
Hard-cooked egg whites—2
Grape tomatoes—6 medium
*Place on a bed of leafy green lettuce.
Use olive oil spray to grill.*
Calories: 430 / Carbs: 30 grams

SNACK OPTIONS

Del Monte light fruit cup—
  4 ounces
Low-fat cottage cheese—
  4 ounces
Calories: 130 / Carbs: 16 grams

_____

All-Bran cereal—½ cup
  (has 10 grams of fiber)
Light fruit yogurt—4 ounces
Calories: 135 / Carbs: 24 grams

_____

Baby carrots—mini bag
Hummus—4 tablespoons
Calories: 155 / Carbs: 22 grams

_____

Blueberries—½ cup
Low-fat cottage cheese—
  4 ounces
Calories: 120 / Carbs: 13 grams

_____

Apple—medium (5½ ounce)
Almonds—6 to 12
*Calories: 140–175 /
Carbs: 23 grams*

_____

Whole wheat mini pita—
  1 ounce
Tomato and lettuce
Feta, reduced fat—1 ounce
Calories: 120 / Carbs: 15 grams

_____

Light yogurt—8 ounces
Calories: 120 / Carbs: 20 grams

_____

Pear—medium (6 ounces)
String cheese—1 ounce
Calories: 150 / Carbs: 22 grams

_____

Wasa light rye crackers—2
Laughing Cow light cheese—
  1 ounce
Calories: 110 / Carbs: 10 grams

_____

Mozzarella, skim—1 ounce
Tomato, sliced—medium
  (5 ounces)
Fresh basil with wine vinegar—
  2 ounces
Calories: 100 / Carbs: 8 grams

_____

Edamame (soybeans)—1 cup
  in pods
Calories: 120 / Carbs: 10 grams

_____

Healthy Choice Garden
  Vegetable Soup—1 cup
Calories: 120 / Carbs: 27 grams

_____

Apple—medium (5½ ounce)
Natural peanut butter—
  1 tablespoon
Calories: 195 / Carbs: 23 grams

_____

Canned lite peaches—½ cup
  (drained)
Low-fat cottage cheese—4 ounces
Calories: 130 / Carbs: 14 grams

_____

Corn tortilla (baked)—6 inches
Low-fat cheese, shredded—
  1 ounce
Salsa—2 tablespoons
Calories: 140 / Carbs: 10 grams

_____

Low-sodium V-8 juice—
  8 ounces
Celery—2 stalks

Tabasco and pepper (optional)
Calories: 60 / Carbs: 10 grams

Popcorn (light)—3 cups
Calories: 75 / Carbs: 12 grams

Bean salad—½ cup (7 grams
of fiber)
Calories: 110 / Carbs: 10 grams

Hard-boiled egg—1
Whole wheat roll—1 ounce
Mustard—1 teaspoon
Calories: 155 / Carbs: 15 grams

Jicama—3 ounces
Red bell peppers—1 medium
(cut into strips)
Light ranch dressing—
2 tablespoons
Calories: 140 / Carbs: 14 grams

Kozy Shack Lite pudding—
4 ounces
Calories: 110 / Carbs: 22 grams

Sugar-free Jell-O—½ cup
Cool Whip Lite—2 tablespoons
Calories: 25 / Carbs: none

Whole wheat mini bagel—
2 ounces
Lox (nova)—2 ounces
Light cream cheese—
2 tablespoons
Calories: 185 / Carbs: 20 grams

Mini pita—1 ounce
Lettuce, cherry tomatoes
Tzatziki (yogurt cucumber
dip)—2 tablespoons
Calories: 115 / Carbs: 15 grams

Cantaloupe—1 cup
Prosciutto—1 ounce
Calories: 125 / Carbs: 13 grams

Pita chips—1 ounce (8 chips)
Tzatziki—2 tablespoons
Calories: 170 / Carbs: 18 grams

Peanuts—1 ounce
Calories: 165 / Carbs: 6 grams

Soy nuts (roasted)—1 ounce
Calories: 130 / Carbs: 9 grams

Celery—2 stalks
Herbed light cream cheese—
2 tablespoons
Calories: 90 / Carbs: 4 grams

Choice Bar—1
Calories: 140 / Carbs: 19 grams

Nite Bite—1
Calories: 100 / Carbs: 15 grams

Pria Bar—1
Calories: 110 / Carbs: 17 grams

Tiger's Milk Bar—1
Calories: 145 / Carbs: 18 grams

Design Your Exercise Plan

1. First you should always check with your physician before starting a program.

2. List three activities you enjoy.

    _____   _____   _____

3. What time of day do you want to exercise? _____

4. What days do you want to exercise on? _____

5. Where are you going to exercise? _____

6. How long are you going to exercise? _____

7. What barriers have prevented you in the past from exercising?

    _____   _____   _____

8. Do you have an alternate exercise plan? Yes _____ No _____

9. What is your alternate plan? _____

10. What are your exercise goals?

    _____   _____   _____

11. List ways to reward yourself without food.

    _____   _____   _____

12. Have fun and enjoy yourself!

Exercise Schedule Log

Cardiovascular

Sunday	Monday	Tuesday	Wednesday	Thursday	Friday	Saturday

Resistance Training

Sunday	Monday	Tuesday	Wednesday	Thursday	Friday	Saturday

Stretching

Sunday	Monday	Tuesday	Wednesday	Thursday	Friday	Saturday

NOTES

1. Isomaa B., P. Almgren, T. Tuomi, B. Forsen, K. Lahti, M. Nissen, et al. 2001. "Cardiovascular morbidity and mortality associated with the metabolic syndrome." *Diabetes Care* 24:683–89. Hu F. B., M. J. Stampfer, S. M. Haffner, C. G. Solomon, W. C. Willett, and J. E. Manson. 2002. "Elevated risk of cardiovascular disease prior to clinical diagnosis of type 2 diabetes." *Diabetes Care* 25 (7):1129–34.
2. Knochenhauer, E. S., T. J. Key, M. Kahsar-Miller, W. Waggoner, L. R. Boots, and R. Azziz. 1998. "Prevalence of the polycystic ovary syndrome in unselected black and white women of the southeastern United States: A prospective study." *Journal of Clinical Endocrinology and Metabolism* 83 (9):3078–82.
3. Jayagopal, V., E. S. Kilpatrick, P. E. Jennings, D. A. Hepburn, and S. L. Atkin. 2003. "The biological variation of testosterone and sex hormone-binding globulin (SHBG) in polycystic ovarian syndrome: Implications for SHBG as a surrogate marker of insulin resistance." *Journal of Clinical Endocrinology and Metabolism* 88 (4):1528–33. Veldhuis, J. D., S. M. Pincus, M. C. Garcia-Rudaz, M. G. Ropelato, M. E. Escobar, and M. Barontini. 2001. "Disruption of the joint synchrony of luteinizing hormone, testosterone, and androstenedione secretion in adolescents with polycystic ovarian syndrome." *Journal of Clinical Endocrinology and Metabolism* 86 (1):72–79. Hopkinson, Z. E., N. Sattar, R. Fleming, and I. A. Greer. 1998. "Polycystic ovarian syndrome: The metabolic syndrome comes to gynaecology." *British Medical Journal* 317 (7154):329–32. Vanky, E., S. Kjatrad, K. A. Salvesen, P. Romundstad, M. H. Moen, and S. M. Carlsen. 2004. "Clinical, biochemical and ultrasonographic characteristics of Scandinavian women with PCOS." *Acta Obstetricia et Gynecologica Scandinavica* 83 (5):482–86.
4. Stadtmauer, L. A., S. K. Toma, R. M. Riehl, and L. M. Talbert. 2001. "Metformin treatment of patients with polycystic ovary syndrome undergoing in vitro fertilization improves outcomes and is associated with modulation of the insulin-like growth factors." *Fertility and Sterility* 75 (3):505–9. McCarthy, E. A., S. P. Walker, K. McLachlan, J. Boyle, and M. Permezel. 2004. "Metformin in obstetric and gynecologic practice: A review." *Obstetrical and Gynecological Survey* 59 (2):118–27.
5. Prochaska, J. O., C. C. DiClemente, and J. C. Norcross. 1992. "In search of how people change: Applications to addictive behaviors." *American Psychologist* 47: 1102–14.

6. Buchanan, T. A., A. H. Xiang, R. K. Peters, S. L. Kjos, A. Morroquin, and J. Goico, et al. 2002. "Preservation of pancreatic beta-cell function and prevention of type 2 diabetes by pharmacological treatment of insulin resistance in high-risk Hispanic women." *Diabetes* 51: 2796–2803. Diabetes Prevention Program Research Group. 2002. "Reduction in the incidence of type 2 diabetes with lifestyle intervention or metformin." *New England Journal of Medicine* 346:393–403. Chiasson, J. L., R. G. Josse, R. Gomis, M. Hanefeld, A. Karasik, and M. Laakso, and the STOP-NIDDM Trial Research Group. 2003. "Acarbose treatment and the risk of cardiovascular disease and hypertension in patients with impaired glucose tolerance: The STOP-NIDDM trial." *Journal of the American Medical Association* 290 (4):486–94.

INDEX